"Invigorating and delightful, Kombucha Phenomenon clearly presents everything you need to know about America's new and popular health tea. To your health!"

—Ray Sahelian, M.D.
Author of *Melatonin: Nature's Sleeping Pill*

"The definitive tea mushroom handbook has arrived! It is written by Sanford Holst and Betsy Pryor, recognized... authority on Kombucha and one of the first to bring it public on a large scale basis in the United States.

—Holistic Health News

"Congratulations for a book about Kombucha written with information based on hands-on experience, integrity, intelligence and a loving spirit."

—Joan Wilen & Lydia Wilen
Authors of *Chicken Soup & Other Folk Remedies*

"Betsy Pryor, the founder of Laurel Farms, said... 'We just want to make sure that people can acquire a safe Kombucha'."

—The New York Times

Kombucha

PHENOMENON

The Miracle Health Tea

How to Safely Make and Use Kombucha

Betsy Pryor & Sanford Holst

SECOND EDITION

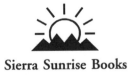

Sierra Sunrise Books

Sierra Sunrise Publishing, Inc.
14622 Ventura Boulevard, Suite 800
Sherman Oaks, California 91403

Printed in the United States of America

First Printing: July, 1995
Second Printing: September, 1995
Third Printing: April, 1996

Publisher's Cataloging-in-Publication Data

Pryor, Betsy
      Kombucha phenomenon : the miracle health tea : how to safely make and
      use kombucha/by Betsy Pryor and Sanford Holst
      p. cm.
      Includes bibliographical references and index.
      ISBN 1-887263-11-X

   1. Tea fungus—Therapeutic use. 2. Medicinal plants. I.
Holst, Sanford. II. Title

RM666.T25P79 1995   615'.321
                          QBI95-20104

Library of Congress Catalog Card Number: 95-72008

Cover design by Jim More, Prototype Graphics, Los Angeles, CA.
Cover Photo by Eric Sander, Los Angeles, CA.

CONTENTS

Introduction 9

1 Miracles: What Kombucha Can and Cannot Do............ 17

    Energy 19
    Skin 20
    Hair 24
    Weight 26
    Muscle 28
    Sex 30
    Diabetes 30
    Multiple sclerosis 34
    Yeast infections 38
    HIV, AIDS 40
    Cancer 42
    Chronic fatigue 45
    Indigestion, ulcers, stress 48
    Migraine, arthritis, rheumatism 50
    Sore throat, colds, flu, allergy, asthma 53
    Other ailments 55
    Seniors' problems 58

2 Safety 61

    Contamination 61
    Protection against contamination 66
    Rumors 68
    Do's and Don'ts 75

3 How to Make Kombucha Tea 77

   Before your mushroom arrives 78
   Here's what you'll need 78
   Substitutions? 82
   The first time you make tea 82
   So let's cook! 83
   After seven to ten days 85
   Now, start again right away 87
   How many mushrooms will you want to keep? 88
   Problems that may come up and
      what to do about them 89
   How to give someone a Kombucha 93
   Herbal tea 94
   When you get a new mushroom 95
   Make a friend 96
   Summary 97

4 Drinking the Tea and Other Uses 101

   Drinking tea the first time 103
   Storing your tea 103
   Kombucha tea in health food stores 105
   Side effects? 106
   How do you feel? 107
   Other uses 107
   Pet and animal uses 109

5 History and Research 115

   China 115
   Japan 116
   Russia 117
   Europe 119
   United States 120

5   History and Research (Continued)

A rose by any other name 122

Holistic health 123

Theories 126

6   What is Kombucha? 129

Technical stuff 129

Combination 130

Mushroom? 131

Fermentation 131

Classification 132

7   References 137

Where to find a Kombucha 137

Information 138

Internet 138

Books and articles 141

8   The Last Word 153

Index 155

NOTE

Although Kombucha is popularly known as a "mushroom" it is actually a healthy combination of bacteria and yeast.

Lipton™, Pyrex™, Anchor-Hocking™, Libby™, Luminarc™, Kombucha Tea™ and Laurel Farms™ are registered trademarks.

The authors make no claims regarding benefits of the Kombucha "mushroom" or tea. Always seek the advice of your health care provider.

INTRODUCTION

Would you like to have a miracle come into your life? Who wouldn't?

It's rare. But it happens. Lotteries have to give the money to *someone*. People with "incurable diseases" have miracle cures. A scientist's room full of electronics are squeezed into a child's Game Boy. If you didn't see it yourself, you wouldn't believe it.

Kombucha seems to be one of those rare miracles. We didn't believe it. But people around us swore by it. Then we tried it. And it became hard *not* to believe.

We didn't stop there. Years of research went into checking hundreds of sources and interviewing thousands of people who use the tea, before we finally got a clear picture of what was going on.

It turns out some of the claims are true. Some aren't. Some ways of preparing the tea are safe. Some aren't.

What happens if you do it wrong? People's reactions range from mild to severe. We've uncovered a wealth of information. Many of these startling discoveries are presented here for the first time.

We discovered there's only one way to make the tea safely with best results. It's shown on the pages that follow.

You'll also see some of the miracles, which people tell in their own words. Their experiences range from simple things like having better skin or losing weight...to people with arthritis in their legs who can walk again, or people with AIDS who see infections go down.

We try to give insights and show why things are happening. But there's something else. And it's hard to put into words. After talking with people who suffered for many years—then recovered their physical abilities and that glad-to-be-alive feeling—sometimes all we could do was go for a long walk and wonder at the miracle of life.

❀   ❀   ❀

Not all new beginnings happen with trumpet fanfares and the singing of angels. For Sandy Holst, it just began with a ringing telephone.

We made a great discovery in 1993—at least, Betsy Pryor did. Kombucha tea.

I got an amazing phone call.

"What if you could improve your life by drinking tea?" she said excitedly.

"I am, Betsy. Lipton's."

"Seriously. This is Kombucha tea."

"Come again?"

"A mushroom you put in tea. The tea ferments a little until it tastes like cider."

"You drink this?"

"Every day. And I feel great! You want to try some?"

"Uh…sure, Betsy. Eventually."

Come on. I'm a guy who exercises every morning. Why would I need a mushroom?

A few months later, another friend called. She was feeling terrific and doing lots of new things. She started telling me about a mushroom.

"You on this Kombucha thing?"

"Yes! Got it from Betsy. Did you get one?"

"Uh…not yet."
Could be just a fad. Probably blow over in a few months.

Then *Los Angeles Magazine* did a fascinating article on people
across the country trying a new tea and claiming remarkable results
that affected all parts of their body. I've always been intrigued by
the holistic, whole-body approach to healing. Spent years collect-
ing books and articles on it. This looked promising. The article was
about Kombucha tea. It talked about Kombucha not being a mushroom—only looked like one. It featured a woman who had distrib-
uted thousands of these "mushrooms." Betsy Pryor.
I picked up the telephone. Had to see a lady about a mushroom.

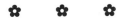

Kombucha tea turned out to be an invigorating health bever-
age that seems to help people in many different ways.
It's used by society leaders and home-makers, active people of
both sexes, bankers and clerks, and older Americans. Celebrities too.
Newspapers and magazines report that Kombucha is used by Daryl
Hannah, Ronald Reagan, Rita Coolidge, Madonna, Sharon Farrell,
Morgan Fairchild, Linda Evans, Graham Russel and Lily Tomlin.
It's spreading like wildfire. The last time this happened was over
a new exercise called "aerobics."
Why the excitement?
To tell the truth, the dramatic results people get from drinking
Kombucha tea are hard to believe. That's why you won't hear it from
us. Instead, we're including a wide sampling of research facts and
people's personal experiences. Decide for yourself.
People say the tea has helped them with migraine, digestion,
skin problems, chemotherapy symptoms, AIDS symptoms, illnesses,

insomnia, regularity, T-cell count, multiple sclerosis remission, asthma, eczema, low energy, wrinkle reduction, restoring some hair color, improving memory, sex drive, cellulite, weight reduction, acne, allergies, PMS, rashes, headaches, rheumatism, arthritis, gallstones, hemorrhoids, gout and bronchitis.

One of the great things about the Kombucha mushroom is that it multiplies as it grows. People often give the new ones to friends so they can make their own tea.

How do you make it? It's fairly easy once you know how. Betsy Pryor's method for preparing Kombucha tea is widely acclaimed as the best and safest way. And "safe" is important. Because it's possible to do it wrong, just like with any other food. All across the country and around the world, people are doing it right. You can too.

Very simply (we go into lots of detail later) a Kombucha mushroom is put into a bowl of tea and sugar. As it grows, the tea ferments. After a week or so, the mushroom is moved to a fresh bowl. Then you drink the mildly-fermented tea.

What's in the tea? Healthy enzymes, organic acids, vitamins and other good things. It's all explained, along with references to long, scientific names that get technical people excited. The "mushroom" that makes the tea is a combination of healthy bacteria and yeast—and though we don't recommend that people eat it, some do. Normally, you just drink the tea.

The story of where Kombucha came from is long and rich with images from many countries, as you will see. The important thing is: what does it do now that it's here?

The excited reactions of people across America reveal the answer. They share their vivid experiences with family members, neighbors, old friends and people they just met. It's the talk of the country.

We'll go into all that.

❀   ❀   ❀

Betsy Pryor describes the journey that made her care about people's health and Kombucha. It began, oddly enough, on a trip to Liberia, West Africa in 1981:

It was early evening. Humid. Hot as hell. Rainy season coming. I sat in the bar of Julia's Hotel in what passed for downtown Monrovia, nursing a Fanta and waiting for a friend to return from flying the body of a local official back to his village deep in the bush. I stared at the spatter of bullet holes crazy-quilted across the wall behind the bar while I listened to the conversation of two American geologists a couple of stools down. They drank local beer and talked about some mysterious thing called the "Black Rose." I leaned closer. Seemed it was a new venereal disease. Left purplish sores that look like rose petals on the limbs of its victims. "A Lebanese bar girl down the street died from it today," one of the guys whispered. I put down my Fanta with a clunk and moved over a stool.

"Died?" I gasped, thinking of the panic that the herpes epidemic was causing among my very hip friends in the TV business in L.A. "From a venereal disease? She died?"

They took another swig of their beer, then nodded in unison. "Yeah. Everybody who gets it dies," one said. "First they get the sores. Then pneumonia. Then…" He made a slicing gesture across his throat. They shook their heads and ordered another round of Club.

I stared blankly up at the ceiling fan slowly slapping against the torpid air, then looked out the open door to the dusty street, where white European and American men, the engineers, geologists and mining experts who populated this far-away place, strolled in the warm African evening with their "special girls." It's over, I thought.

All over. Those guys would go back to the States. Infect their wives. Their girlfriends. I closed my eyes.

I never forgot that night. It was marked on my soul with an indelible blot. By 1983, the "Black Rose" had been given a name. AIDS. Late at night I would lie awake wondering what had happened to the American and European men and their "special girls." How many of the "girls" were dead? How many of the men had brought the disease back home? And what about the blood bankers who'd come to town that muggy African January so long ago, trolling for cheap blood. How many units did they buy? How many were tainted with the yet-to-be-detected virus? Where did those units end up? Who, I wondered, had they infected?

Already a technical writer, I began studying viruses, talking to scientists, physicists and physicians. Off the record, they told me that what we had seen so far was a walk in the park compared to what was to come. My instincts were right, they confided. Because we live in a toxic environment, people's immune systems were weakening. Viruses and bacteria would mutate. Become deadly, even airborne. By the year 2010, we could be looking at the end of the human race.

In the summer of 1993, exhausted from four years of hard writing on a science thriller about a runaway retrovirus, I had taken to meditating a couple of nights a week with the Brahma Kumaris, a non-governmental organization of the United Nations. One night at class. I silently prayed, "God, please give me *something, anything* to help people stay well."

A few minutes later, as I was leaving, Sister Joan Derry, one of the meditation teachers, bustled out of the kitchen carrying a pancake type thing enclosed in a clear, plastic bag. "Wait," she called, her cherubic face split in a wide grin, "I've got something for you!"

The thing in the bag looked awful. I backed away. "What," I whispered, "*is* it?"

"It's a Kombucha tea mushroom! People drink the tea it makes, and they *feel* better." She handed me a faded sheet of paper. "Look at all the stuff it's good for!"

I scanned the sheet. Fixes everything from arthritis to acne to acid stomach to a hundred other things, it said. I handed it back to her. "Snake oil," I declared, having spent the last three years in medical libraries. "*Nothing* can do all that. Except God."

"Take the Kombucha anyway. Sister Denise and I decided that if anybody was going to get it out to people, it was going to be you."

"Yeah, right," I thought as I walked out into the night.

After two weeks of drinking Kombucha tea, the acne I'd had since age 13 was gone. I'd also lost the first of the 15 pounds I'd put on since high school. I had to admit I looked and felt pretty good.

And since the Kombucha makes a "baby mushroom" every week, in a few months I'd given one to each neighbor on our little canyon cul-de-sac. Everybody else was feeling pretty good, too. Gates and fences were being mended and painted for the first time in a dozen years. My neighbor Joe, who had just turned 71, was spending a lot of time three stories in the air repairing his roof. A second neighbor was spending Sundays hanging off the side of the cliff edging her property, chopping at the brush with a machete. She was 65 and starting to look a lot like Doris Day. Another neighbor was showing off the black hairs creeping back into his graying ponytail. I thought I was watching the sequel to *Cocoon*.

I had to admit. The stuff was working. All right, so I hadn't found a cure for AIDS. But I *did* find something that was helping people keep healthy. And had to do something about it.

In January of 1994, I took Joan and Denise's advice. It *was* time to get Kombucha to people. Three days after the Los Angeles earthquake, I started Laurel Farms—and began sending Kombucha mushrooms all across the country.

Later came the TV, radio, newspaper and magazine excitement. We were on our way.

MIRACLES: WHAT KOMBUCHA CAN AND CANNOT DO

An amazing number of health improvements have been claimed for Kombucha. They overflow from published articles and TV programs. They're printed in long lists on information sheets handed from person to person—copied so many times the original authors are unknown. Are all of these claims true? No.

But a surprisingly large number of them are true—verified by person after person describing similar results. As you'll see.

Unfortunately, some of the claims are outrageous, and out of all the people we've interviewed, no one has confirmed them. Those claims cause some people to shake their heads and assume that Kombucha doesn't work at all. Very unfortunate.

What are some of the misleading claims? One woman says it helped her friend grow back part of his ear. Come on. Many people report that it clears up skin rashes, psoriasis and burns. But grow an ear?

Another widespread claim is that Kombucha cures cancer. We wish it was true. Too many people are still suffering from cancer. It's not a cure. On the other hand, it may assist in cancer treatment. People going through difficult chemotherapy have reported Kombucha helps their body rebound from the after-effects and get back to normal more quickly.

To compile the information shown on the following pages, we talked with literally thousands of people who use Kombucha. Many of their experiences were documented in writing, and are included here. Taken together, they form a clearer picture of what Kombucha can and cannot do than has ever been published before.

Why do this? Because we're not allowed to make health claims. Although there have been many studies performed in other countries over the past hundred years (see the History chapter), American medical practice doesn't recognize them. It is widely estimated that the extensive tests required for certification in the U.S. cost hundreds of millions of dollars. Drug companies normally pay those costs. Why do that? Because their new products can be brought to market at prices that produce billions of dollars in revenue. For them, it's good business.

One problem. Kombucha is free. Since each Kombucha makes a second "mushroom" every 7–10 days, people give them away to family and friends. True, if you don't know someone with an extra Kombucha, you can buy one from a commercial grower. But we estimate over 90% of the three million people in the U.S. who use Kombucha got it free from someone they know.

So. Without millions of dollars to spend on extensive testing, what can we do? Just exactly what we're doing. Collect the information and get it out as widely as possible. Let people make up their minds. In talking with folks all over the country, we've found that most Americans have a lot of common sense. They look at things carefully and then decide for themselves.

People who use—and swear by—Kombucha tea come from all walks of life. Their health before trying this experience varied all over the map. Some were in reasonably good shape and wanted to get better. Others had very difficult problems—including multiple sclerosis or AIDS—and were looking for anything to give them a chance. We can't give medical opinions. We're not doctors, and it wouldn't be fair to try.

The people quoted here tell their own experiences. They come from South Bend, Indiana and Boca Raton, Florida. From New York

City and Los Angeles. From Seattle and Berryville, Arkansas. They come from cities and towns all across America. Maybe yours.

In the following section we look at the full list of health improvements associated with Kombucha. And include comments by doctors, natural health practitioners and people who actually experienced the improvements.

The key to understanding these things—and what happens when you drink the tea—requires some understanding of what your whole body is doing. This a key part of holistic health. First we'll look at the individual health problems that Kombucha seems to help, then we'll look at what causes the effect, and how it all comes together.

Take a look at the following facts and experiences...and decide for yourself.

ENERGY

The first thing reported by almost everyone who drinks this special tea is that they have more energy. For example, Joe in Los Angeles says, "In a couple of days, I had such energy—and I'm 71. I can do heavy work now if I want to, and I take care of things around the house, like paint and repair the roof."

John in New York City adds, "General spirit, attitude and energy was very low. After one week of drinking the tea, all these improved. I have much more stamina."

There are different opinions on why this happens. Some people point out that the ingredients used in making the tea contain caffeine and sugar—and they guess that the energy is just a "hit" of stimulants. Not so, say researchers who have studied the processes in detail.

Their studies show that the caffeine and sugar are almost entirely used up during the 7–10 day process of growing the mushroom and making the Kombucha tea. As a result, caffeine and sugar are present in only small amounts in the Kombucha beverage that you actually drink. Dr. Bruker reported in 1986, "After 10 days, the starting sugar has long since been fermented." Early in this process, refined sugar is broken down into simple sugar called glucose. Dr. Reiss added in 1987, "Around the 17th day, the reserves of glucose are nearly exhausted."

Kombucha tea appears to have several beneficial effects that add up to more energy. First, it seems to aid digestion. The drink is slightly acidic, like the juices in your stomach, which can help to start the digestive process. We measured the pH (acidity) of the tea and found it to be in the range of 3.5 to 2.0 during the growing process. This confirmed earlier measurements by Dr. Reiss. Kombucha tea also contains healthy bacteria believed to work with the natural bacteria in our digestive tract, which frees the food's nutrients to be picked up by the bloodstream. Finally, the tea contains glucuronic acid, which helps the liver and kidneys extract toxins from your body and move them out of the system as waste. We'll talk more about glucuronic acid later.

So where does the extra energy come from?

From your food. Better digestion moves the nutrients into your bloodstream so that it goes to all parts of your body. And as more toxins are removed from your system, your body doesn't have to keep fighting them and can put the nutrients to good use—letting you stay active longer.

SKIN

One of the best windows into a person's health is their skin. It can be smooth, elastic and soft to the touch. Or it can have rashes, blotches, wrinkles and sag a little more each year. Many people say, "Of course those lousy things happen. You're just getting older." Not so.

Have you ever noticed some people age much better than others? And some teenagers go through huge bouts of acne while others don't?

The most common remedies for these conditions is to put lotion on the skin. If it's very serious, some doctors write prescriptions for stronger lotions.

No offense intended, but that's like fixing wood that has dry rot by giving it a coat of paint. Temporarily it looks better. What's been cured?

The healthier, holistic approach is to fix the many parts of the body that work together to produce good skin. Kombucha seems to help the body do that.

What produces healthy skin? We don't want to get too bogged down in technical terms, but there are a couple of things you ought to know.

What you see as "skin" is just the surface layer. Doctors call it the epidermis. It's fairly tough and not very thick. Under it is a second skin layer called the dermis where the real action happens. The dermis is laced with blood vessels, nerves, sweat glands and the base of each strand of hair. This is where fresh skin is made.

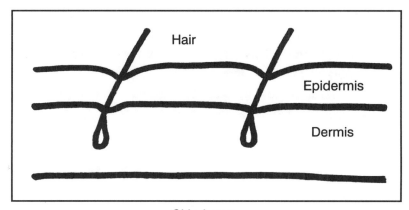

Skin layers

When all's working well, the dry, tough, cracked surface skin wears away and is replaced by the fresh, smooth skin that grows underneath. If you want a quick demonstration, go watch someone with sunburn. Part of the top layer peels off in a couple of days.

Doctors sometimes accelerate this process by physically removing part of the top layer of skin in processes called "dermabrasion," peels, and laser reduction. A standard beauty treatment called "loofah" accomplishes a similar purpose by using a rough sponge to scrub off top skin. But if the skin that grows to replace it is also in poor condition, what's been accomplished?

If your body is not really healthy, the new layer is not as smooth, not as elastic as when you were a kid. Want proof? What happens when you get a cut on your finger?

When you're a kid, it scabs up right away, the next day or two the scab falls off, and a couple of days later you can't see where the cut was. From your twenties onward it takes a little longer to heal, then longer, then it never quite goes away—leaving a white or red mark where the cut happened. Why?

Because many parts of your body have to work well and contribute the right materials for healing and repairing your skin. Good blood flow is a major factor, and requires a healthy heart, arteries that aren't clogged with fatty tissue, and healthy lungs that get oxygen into the blood. A good liver and kidneys are needed to take waste products out of the blood, a good digestive system is needed to put nutrients in. A healthy nerve system is needed to send the proper signals to guide the process.

If any one of these isn't working, where are you? When all of them work poorly, what do you think happens?

If Kombucha works the way we believe it does—improving digestion, helping the liver get rid of toxins, providing vitamins, necessary organic acids and other nutrients—what do you think would happen to the different parts of your body? To your skin?

Several people from around the country describe what happened to them when they drank Kombucha tea.

Norma from Holbrook, Massachusetts says, "My skin, especially my face, has become tighter and younger looking. I have more energy. I don't have that tired feeling when I get up in the a.m., and I can stay up longer at night. I almost forgot, my hair has thickened all over. I have received a lot of compliments about my skin [and] hair."

Rashes, wrinkles and sagging are not the only skin problems that can occur. Acne and excess oil can become serious problems. Martha in Amarillo, Texas describes her experience.

"I am 47 years old. I have had a very bad complexion problem since I was about 12 or 13 years old—which was mostly caused by an extreme excess of oil in the skin on my face which I could not get rid of. I have been to several dermatologists and have had everything from antibiotics, creams and medications (including Accutane and Retin-A), all kinds of restricted diets, dry ice, X-ray, and finally last year I had a dermabrasion on my face. Nothing helped. The dermabrasion somewhat helped the looks, because it smoothed out the scars. However, it did not get rid of the root of the problem—the oil, which was a great disappointment to me.

"This is something I have battled for 34 years. I had decided it was hopeless. The oil was so bad that I could wash my face until the outer layer was so dry it would peel, but 30 minutes later I could rub my fingers across my forehead or cheek and they would literally be shiny and slick with the oil from my face. It was a mess needless to say. Not only was it so oily, but my face was always red and irritated looking.

"I have been drinking the mushroom tea now for 2½ months and I am very, very pleased with the results I am having with my body. For the first time since becoming a teenager the *excess oil is completely gone* from my face!! This is a miracle!

"Between myself and the insurance companies, we have spent thousands of dollars trying to solve a problem that could have been so simply and quickly solved years ago had I known about the mushroom tea. I know beyond a shadow of a doubt it is the tea that has dried the oil from my skin.

"I began noticing a change after drinking it for about 2 weeks. At first I thought it was my imagination or that, as many times before, it would seemingly dry out a little for 2 or 3 days but then the oil would always come back. It was not my imagination! The excess oil has been totally and completely gone now for 2 full months. Not only is all the oil gone, but my face is not red and irritated looking any more. It is clear and normal except for scars for the first time since puberty. I am so excited and happy! I have gotten many compliments the past few weeks on the change in my complexion. I intend to drink this tea for the rest of my life."

So. Will Kombucha or anything else repair all the damage that has happened to your body over many years? Probably not. But Kombucha seems to make such a significant improvement for many people that others notice.

Martin Landau was reported on the E! cable channel news to have seen a movie director at lunch and complimented the man on his new facelift. The director replied that he didn't have a facelift—he was drinking Kombucha tea! So Martin Landau got a Kombucha mushroom for himself.

Hey, guys like to look good too.

Leo, a bartender in Cedar Rapids, Iowa describes his experience this way. "I have shared the strange little things with a lot of people. I have noticed much success with them all. The greatest thing I have noticed is how it helps in digestion and also much improved skin.

"A few months ago [my nutritionist] said, 'Leo I saw this product at a conference…. It was like God taking me by the hand.' She is a wonderful woman and I am sold on [the] mushroom."

HAIR

When we first heard people comment about what Kombucha does for their hair, we were more than a little skeptical. Make white or gray hair go back to its original color? Cause hair to be thicker and fuller? Come on.

Boy, were we wrong. One of the most frequent comments we get from people with white or gray hair is that they get dark roots—

and then the darker hair just keeps growing out. Not just black, but also brown, blond or whatever color it was originally. You have to see it to believe it. Betsy was getting some gray. It went away. We believe it.

Not everyone is happy about the change. Some older folks with beautiful platinum hair started getting salt-and-pepper and didn't want it. Others were delighted.

Rose of Santa Ana, California says, "After using the mushroom [tea] for about three days I realized…I had much more energy and more things were getting done around the house. I have about 125 orchids which I do myself, and I live on a third of an acre. I had a two inch band of snow white hair surrounding my face. I now have brown hair on the top of my head. On the two sides by my ears it's still a little bit gray, but not much!"

Rose's experience gives you a clue as to why this happens.

Kombucha is not like most traditional medicines which target one specific thing—like cough medicine for a sore throat, or anti-biotics for a viral infection. Kombucha seems to help all the different parts of your body work normally. Then your body heals itself.

Think about it. Who is born with white hair? Is that normal? No. Normal hair has melanin for color and other materials to make it full and strong. As years go by, your arteries start taking hits from cholesterol, then liquor does a number on your liver, your lungs labor from smoke and debris in the air—they no longer support each other as well as they used to.

Each hair grows out of a follicle in the skin. And we talked about the skin already—if it's not getting the support it needs from the rest of the body, what happens to the hair it makes?

Right. Melanin production goes down and the new hair grows out gray. A few trips to the barber or hairdresser, and your dark hair is on the floor. You've joined the gray panthers.

You can get your hair dyed, of course. And many people do. It's a temporary fix that you have to do over and over. Does that cure anything?

So what's the miracle with Kombucha and hair? No miracle. When the rest of your body works right, your skin can make healthy hair—the same color it was before.

Deepak Chopra made an excellent point in his book *Ageless Body, Timeless Mind.* Your genes contain all the blueprints to make a body as healthy as when you were young. If you have the right attitude and physical materials, your body is capable of repairing itself.

A hairstylist named William in Akron, Ohio drinks the tea and uses it externally. He describes his experience this way. "I can't say enough about the Kombucha tea, it's help[ed] me in many ways. My days are more productive.... I have scars on my face, it has taken the red out. I use it in [the] morning to freshen and tighten my adult face. I've lost 15 lb from the tea.

"I use it (mushroom tea) in my hair as a rinse. It seems to have strengthen[ed] my hair; not so much hair is falling out. Plus I have friends that can't do without it now."

WEIGHT

This is one of the most visible changes reported by people who drink Kombucha tea. And it has one of the most remarkable effects: it seems to help people get back to the weight that's right for them—whether that means adding weight or losing it.

Wait a minute, you say. What does "the weight that's right for them" mean? It means the chart on the doctor's wall that says how much a man or woman should weigh, based on their height.

Don't know about you, but our reaction to those charts was always, "No way." A person would be *skinny* at those weights. Right? At least that's the excuse we used for being a bit overweight.

A personal experience by Sandy Holst. "I looked in the mirror when I was shaving one morning and said, 'Oh no. Looks like I'm getting sick.' Strange. I had been drinking the tea for several months and hadn't been sick in a long time. I felt OK, but my face looked thinner—like a person who has a bug of some kind and is wasting away.

"I checked the scale. I'd lost ten pounds. Stranger still. Ever since I got out of school and took one desk job after another, I had been fifteen pounds over the doctors' charts. I'd always figured, what the heck—everyone in America is fifteen pounds overweight. That made my weight normal...sort of. Now it wasn't.

"I worried for a few days. But didn't come down with a flu or anything. My weight leveled off at fourteen pounds down. And it's stayed close to that level ever since. The really odd thing was that I hadn't done anything different—just drank the tea."

The truly amazing part is that Kombucha also seems to help people *gain* weight if they're below the "correct weight." Before you say something like, "What funny stuff have these people been smoking," consider this experience from Kenneth Sikorsky in Berryville, Arkansas.

"My neighbor's brother has cancer. He lost all his hair and was down to skin and bones. The doctors gave him 6 months to live. His mother got a tea mushroom from someone and he drank the tea for 6 months. Now he has gained 100 lbs and has a full head of hair. The doctors are growing [their] own tea mushroom trying to figure it out."

Those of us who grew up with traditional medicine have some trouble understanding how this is possible. One lunch partner who heard about the weight loss told us, "It's obviously just a diuretic—makes your body artificially get rid of fluids." Another person listened to the weight gain story and concluded the tea has an appetite stimulant which causes people to eat more.

They were reflecting the traditional medicine approach. Give specific medicine to make the body do a specific thing. The concept of just bringing your body into balance seems to have been lost somewhere.

How can one beverage make you gain weight or lose it?

Easy. The tea isn't doing anything about your weight. Your body is. When your body starts getting the right nutrients and rids itself of toxic materials, it begins to adjust back to natural levels of hormone secretion, enzyme production, blood flow, etc.—and your insides start working normally. That's not normally as in "average American." It means normally as in "healthy." Normal weight, normal energy and everything else.

Does this mean Kombucha is going to make everyone the same? No. But it does seem to help people move a little closer to normal. As in healthy.

Gayle of Atlanta, Georgia tells her experience.

"As an obese woman, I have tried every diet known to man and my book shelves groan with the books I have bought to make an attempt to lose weight. I have also tried *all* of the commercial programs, several of them multiple times.

"Since I started the tea, I have reduced one blouse size and three, almost four jeans sizes. In fact, I can now shop at any regular store that has a plus size department. I have a long way to go but, for the first time, I feel that I have taken two steps forward instead of three steps back.

"I don't know how many pounds I have lost. I have decided not to be a slave to numbers. I know where I was when I started; when I get to a reasonable size, I will borrow a scale. I threw mine away several years ago."

MUSCLE

Dr. Boris Wydoff was one of the Soviet physicians who worked with Olympic athletes from 1976 to 1979. He identified Kombucha as one of the reasons their teams were so dominant.

"I was a medical doctor...specialist in sports medicine, to treat people without drugs and surgery. I usually trained athletes in track and field...for the Olympic teams.

"I utilized also alternative, holistic medicines...a combination of things, not one thing.... Some take 4 ounces [of Kombucha], some take 4 ounces three times, some 4 ounces six times a day.... More vitality, more energy, better performance....

"[Kombucha brings] normalization of friendly bacteria in the intestines, and all the B-complex and B vitamins, B_{12} especially, improve in the blood system.... And you know vitality and defense mechanisms depend on the friendly bacteria. And the friendly bacteria thrive in the beverage of Kombucha mushroom tea...."

"To balance the ratio between the weight and muscle.... More vitality, better metabolism. Better metabolism, all the food will burn much faster and the fat cells also. It works all together, our system interdependent on each other.

"This is like better fuel for our blood, the Kombucha mushroom tea because it contains enzymes, vitamins...and glucuronic acid which...is number one for improving the metabolism."

Other people have similar experiences. One reflection of improved muscle tone is the number of people who talk of being able to do hard work they haven't done in years (as seen in other sections).

Some people directly report improvements in muscle tone and firmness. Betsy is one. As she said to Maury Povitch on his TV show, "Feel that muscle!" She held up her arm and he gave her biceps a squeeze, nodding appreciatively.

Then she added, "Feel that thigh!" He looked at her in shock, as if imagining divorce papers being served by his wife, Connie Chung. Betsy didn't let him off that easily. She assured him she did no workouts, just drank the tea. But he had to confirm the result. He finally gave her thigh muscle a squeeze, nodding quite a bit this time.

P.S.—Connie seemed to accept it as part of his job. But if he does it again....

SEX

It's amazing how many people ask, "Does Kombucha improve your sex life?" We'd like to give a good answer for that, but there doesn't seem to be any accepted way to measure it.

We have found, however, that there are a number of related things that seem to improve.

Men report fewer prostate problems.

Women report fewer "female problems" including PMS.

And Peter from Charlotte, North Carolina tells us, "Did you know it improves sexual function? Beats me, but it was an unexpected effect both times I first drank it. Now I'm getting used to it. Seems most prominent if one drinks a lot at one time."

Then there's the combined effect of all the things we've mentioned so far. Better skin, better hair, less weight, firmer muscles, more energy. If it doesn't improve someone's sex life, a lot of good things are going to waste.

We can just imagine a couch-potato husband being told, "Don't ask why, just drink it."

DIABETES

This is a medical disorder that is usually inherited. Surprisingly, Kombucha seems to have a role to play here, as we'll see.

The physical symptoms—weight loss, excessive thirst, damage to blood vessels and sometimes blindness—can now be largely controlled by taking insulin or changing one's diet. It usually occurs when a person's pancreas does not produce enough insulin, which results in very high levels of sugar in the bloodstream.

Although diabetes is rarely a killer once a person gets onto a treatment plan, dealing with it can completely change their life. Strictly controlled diet becomes a serious, every-meal, every-day thing. And measuring blood sugar regularly is critical to making sure the right balance of food and drugs is being maintained. The American Diabetes Association recommends insulin-dependent people check their blood sugar at least four times a day.

For information on diabetes:
American Diabetes Association
1660 Duke Street
Alexandria, VA 22314
(800) 232-3472

The misunderstanding we previously mentioned about sugar in Kombucha is obviously very important to people with diabetes who have to avoid high-sugar foods. It should be pointed out that repeated laboratory analysis shows only a small amount of sugar in the finished tea.

As early as 1928, Dr. Mollenda in Germany found, "Those persons afflicted with diabetes can, according to the expert opinion of doctors, drink well-fermented Kombucha as well as sour milk or sour cream, because the sugar, which for the most part is contained in the tea, is broken down into its component parts and converted by the process of fermentation."

This is confirmed by the results people get from drinking the tea. Alphonse and Evelyn in Perkasie, Pennsylvania both have diabetes. He describes their experience this way.

"My wife started on the Kombucha tea about three weeks ago. She is definitely more energized by the tea, and her diabetes daily testing shows an amazing decrease in her blood sugar content. I'm sure she will have to reduce her insulin strength or switch to oral medicine.

"I too, have diabetes and am experiencing an improvement in my blood sugar and an increase of energy. I test my blood sugar once a day. I have a specialist who says an acceptable range is 70 to

140 if you can keep it there. I was ranging 135-170 over the last six months. I'm looking at a range now between 120-140. My wife's range used to be similar to mine, or higher. She's between 90-120.

"Just the other day I took it over to a woman's house to show her how to use it. She had a group that meets regularly and asked me to talk to them. I sing in a barbershop quartet, and have since 1948. So I don't mind being in front of people.

"We are harvesting four batches tomorrow (8 mushrooms coming out), with four new users."

Adds wife Evelyn, "I haven't felt this well in twenty years."

The American Diabetes Association identifies two kinds of diabetes.

Type I is a severe form of diabetes in which insulin production in the pancreas is impaired, usually resulting in dependence on external doses of insulin, and typically occurring before the age of twenty five. This is normally treated with insulin shots, diet and exercise.

> The health associations listed in these sections contributed valuable information to this book. However they have not conducted independent tests using Kombucha and cannot make recommendations on its use.

Type II is a mild form of diabetes which usually occurs in adults and is characterized by diminished tissue sensitivity to insulin and sometimes by impaired pancreas function, which may be made worse by excess body weight. It is usually treatable by diet, exercise and weight loss. Sometimes diabetes pills or insulin shots are required.

Kombucha is not a cure for diabetes. However, it may help the body produce more of the insulin it needs, allowing a person to reduce their dependence on insulin pills and shots.

CAUTION FOR DIABETICS

Remember—sugar put into the tea when a fresh batch is made will *gradually* be used up during the 7–10 days that the Kombucha takes to make a new mushroom and produce finished tea. If you drink tea that has been grown for less than seven days, substantial amounts of sugar may remain. To be on the safe side, we recommend you grow it closer to ten days. Some people even let it go fourteen days—but then the taste is quite strong and you'll probably want to mix it with distilled water before drinking to make it go down easier.

If you have diabetes and want to try Kombucha, we also recommend that you start with smaller amounts and gradually build up. In addition, you should have one of the small devices that lets you test your own blood sugar (called a glucose monitor), check it regularly, and stop drinking the tea if anything gets out of control. Finally, tell your health care provider that you are drinking the tea.

If he or she is like many doctors across the country, they'll say something like, "Tea? Humbug!" Then they'll follow that with, "It's probably just a coincidence, but your sugar levels are better. Let's decrease your insulin a little."

Most important: do not cut back on your insulin without the consent of your health care provider. If you feel you're doing better, and your body might be getting too much insulin, get a second opinion. Never cut off the insulin by yourself.

Another diabetes experience is told by Laura in Cleveland, Ohio. "I have asthma and was hospitalized for 23 days in Sept., 1995. I was treated with a steroid called prednisone. It causes diabetes by elevating the glucose level in some people, of which I am unfortunate to be one.

"I went into the hospital with a normal glucose level of 80. Two days later it was over 400. I left the hospital insulin dependent and taking oral diabetes medicine, along with the other side effects such as rapid, pounding heartbeat and personality change.

"I know a woman in San Antonio, Texas, and she told me about Kombucha tea, saying it will cure your diabetes. I said to her, 'Oh really,' and to myself, 'yeah right!' But I figured it couldn't hurt so I went to the health food store and bought a quart. Three days later another quart. Three days later, no more insulin shots! One week later no more oral medication for diabetes!

"I know for a fact that it's due to Kombucha because last year I went through the same thing and it took *5 months* to get off diabetes medicine.

"I bought 6 quarts before my friend sent me a culture. I now have 8 that I keep making tea with, and I have given 10 people mushrooms. Each one of them is so thrilled and excited about their personal results."

MULTIPLE SCLEROSIS

Often referred to as "MS," this is a devastating disease which attacks the central nervous system. Its effects can range from blurred vision, poor coordination or bladder problems to actual paralysis. It can strike at any age, but often in young adulthood.

The National Multiple Sclerosis Society says over 330,000 Americans suffer from this disease. About a third of them lose the ability to walk, while many others require a cane or walker.

The MS Society revealed two startling facts—at least startling to us. The cause of MS is not known. And there is no known cure.

As our research continued, we realized this is a pattern. For a number of major diseases that attack and destroy lives, the medical community knows of no cause and no cure. Besides multiple sclerosis, this is true of chronic fatigue, most types of arthritis and other diseases.

We used to feel a little defensive about the fact that Kombucha tea seems to help people who have these diseases—but we didn't know exactly how it worked.

Now we take the other view. How could the medical community and caregivers *not* embrace something like this if it works? Until something better comes along, Kombucha "mushrooms" should be available at every doctor's office in the country.

OK, we'll get off the soapbox.

Since there is no cure, traditional medical treatment for MS usually involves medications to relieve some of the symptoms. This is sometimes combined with physical therapy, diet, rest and counseling to decrease emotional stress.

Kombucha tea is not a cure for MS. However, virtually all the people who have shared their experiences with us report amazing improvements in their physical abilities.

For example, Lupe in West Covina, California, was diagnosed with MS in 1992. Friends always described her as an active and energetic young woman. Then she started to become exhausted doing simple tasks and losing coordination. She consulted doctor after doctor and was given a variety of answers. Finally the tests agreed on the diagnosis she didn't want to hear. Multiple sclerosis.

She and her husband worked to support their family. Now she faced no longer being able to work, with medical bills piling up...Lupe describes it this way.

"I had slowly been feeling the effects of the disease progressing. I did not have the stamina to stand on my feet longer than fifteen minutes, let alone walk for ten minutes. My handwriting had gotten worse, sometimes I could not even hold a pen in my hands.

"In May of 1995 a friend told me about Kombucha and showed me two articles regarding the tea. I told her I was willing to try anything. A couple weeks later she instructed me on the care and preparation of making the tea. I followed the instructions carefully and have been drinking the tea since.

"I can honestly tell you that I have been feeling extremely well. I can stand on my feet for hours at a time. My handwriting has improved tremendously. I can run a couple of blocks. My entire family is now drinking Kombucha and they have felt the energizing effects of the tea."

We do not recommend abandoning traditional medicine and treatments. Future breakthroughs based on these practices may lead to an eventual cure.

However, to strengthen your body and give you back some of the energy and ability that makes life worth living, Kombucha tea may be a good companion for traditional medicine. If you drink the tea, be sure to tell your health care provider so they can consider it in their prescriptions and treatments.

For information on MS:
National Multiple Sclerosis Society
733 3rd Avenue
New York, NY 10017
(800) 344-4867

One more experience with MS. Nancy Henshall is a remarkable woman who brightens the world around her despite, or perhaps because of, what she has seen in it.

"I have MS—was diagnosed in April of '89. I went from using a cane—to a 4-prong cane—to a walker, which I am using now. I…had been unable to take regular steps with my walker, and HAD (past tense!) been bent over the walker, as I 'scooted' along!

"I began drinking my tea in the 1st week-and-a-half of December [1994]. By the time my son came home for the holidays, from Ft. Benning, Georgia, on the 17th of December, the exhaustion that came along with the MS was letting up on me. By Christmas Day, when we went to my cousins house—there was such a welcome change in my mobility!!! In her words, 'You ran up the sidewalk!'

"Of course I didn't literally run—but I was straight up, and taking step-after-step-after-step with my walker!! I am now doing so many things I have been unable to do for 1½–2 years—and feel so much better than I have, in every bit that length of time!!

"I have no other medication—or anything else that I take, other than the Kombucha tea I have been taking, that could account for my doing, and feeling, so very much better!!

"For every bit the length of time I mentioned, I have not been able to, myself alone, make dinner for my family, or make any 'treats' for them because I couldn't get a cake batter from the mixing bowl to the pan. It sounds like such a simple thing—unless, after years of being a wife and mom who has always enjoyed doing this, and more, for my family, you all of a sudden can no longer do 'the simple things.'

"What a thrill—no, what a true blessing, it is to be able to do these things again! I surprised my wonderful husband with, what to most, would be a simple batch of brownies….The best part of the whole thing—I was able to do everything myself!! I was so happy to have a "Momma's Surprise" warm out of the oven for my husband—for the first time in years!!

"I can't tell you how much… regaining an ability that has been 'lost' means to the person and their family—to actually be able to do things that you thought would never be a part of you again!"

YEAST INFECTIONS

This topic ranks high on our often-asked-questions list. People hear that Kombucha contains some varieties of yeast and immediately assume it's bad for people with yeast infections. And potentially fatal for people with weakened immune systems. Even some doctors say this. Not so!

The first and most obvious reason is that "yeast" infections are not caused by common yeast. They're caused by candida. One particular infection caused by candida is called vaginitis. This infection produces a white discharge with a "yeasty" odor. Hence the popular expression "yeast infection."

We describe in the "What is Kombucha?" chapter how every living thing is classified into large groups, then those large groups are divided into smaller groups. One thing that contributes to people's confusion on this subject is that there is a large group called Eumycota. Candida and molds belong to this large group. And so do yeasts. But when this large catch-all is divided into smaller groups …candida, molds and yeasts fall into completely separate groups.

And there is a big difference. Candida and molds reproduce by making spores and have undesirable properties.

Yeasts reproduce by budding or fission, and live by changing sugar into other materials.

Once you know that, things start to make sense.

Candida causes several medical problems, including athlete's foot, vaginitis and thrush (candida albicans). It would make sense to not expose someone with a weakened immune system to destructive organisms such as molds. The mold spores might well generate infections.

But if the above points are true, and they are, there is no logical reason why Kombucha should cause a problem for someone with candida.

It also explains why people like Mike in Sierra Madre, California have experiences like this.

"I have been using/drinking the Kombucha tea 3 weeks and my athlete's foot and acne [have] cleared up! My mom's arthritis is going away. Amazing stuff!"

Spores are small, self-contained units that act like seeds. When placed in the proper conditions, they grow into organisms that put out more spores.

On the other hand, budding yeasts grow by forming a bulge on the side of a yeast cell, the cell nucleus divides, and the new cell divides itself off from the original, forming a branching chain. This group is called saccharomyces, and all yeasts in Kombucha are of this type except for one which is shown below.

Fission yeasts grow by forming a wall across the middle of the cell and then splitting into two new cells. This group is called schizosaccharomyces, and the member of this group which is found in Kombucha is Schizosaccharomyces pombe.

So. With that out of the way let's look at a couple of the other rumors that worry people with weakened immune systems. Some people claim Kombucha readily grows mold like Aspergillus. If true, that would be a real concern. It's not true. As you'll see in the "Safety" chapter, Kombucha has better protection against mold than almost anything in your kitchen. If you make Kombucha right, you should never see mold.

The second alarming rumor is that Kombucha is an antibiotic. Antibiotics can be very effective fighting a particular disease, but can also leave your body's defenses weakened and likely to get other diseases. In the "Safety" chapter we go into more detail about Kombucha, but for now just be aware that the tea's natural ingredients have a mild anti-bacterial effect. That's it. No antibiotics.

Oddly enough, even some people in the AIDS community don't seem to understand these basic concepts. The stakes are high. It's worthwhile for people to take a couple of minutes to understand it.

Bret is a truck driver in Mesa, Arizona.

"I have AIDS. In one month, my candida is gone, I'm gaining weight again, and I've been able to do yard work a couple hours a day. I wouldn't be surprised if my T-cells went up. I was almost bed ridden, now I'm running around everywhere, enjoying life again."

HIV, AIDS

Everyone knows the terrible toll AIDS has taken among friends, acquaintances, the famous, the newborn. Men, women and children.

The World Health Organization reports that since the AIDS epidemic started in the late 1970s, more than 20 million people have been infected with HIV. And over 4.5 million cases of full-blown AIDS have occurred.

What about a cure? There isn't one yet.

As most people know by now, AIDS is caused by a virus known as human immunodeficiency virus (HIV). AIDS is characterized by a defect in natural immunity against disease. People who have it are likely to get serious illnesses which would not be a threat to anyone whose immune system was functioning normally.

The most common of these diseases are Pneumocystis carinii pneumonia (PCP), a parasitic infection of the lungs. And Kaposi's sarcoma, a type of cancer.

Is Kombucha the cure? No.

Can it help? Consider the following.

With AIDS, the sum of all the layers of virus protection in a person's body becomes weakened.

All of the previous sections suggest that Kombucha may help the various parts of your body function more like they did when you were younger and in good health. It won't reverse HIV, but it may help fight off infections.

For information on HIV, AIDS:
Centers for Disease Control
and Prevention (CDC)
[No street address required]
Atlanta, GA 30333
(404) 639-3311

A cure for HIV and AIDS is still needed. But the stronger and healthier a person's body is, the better their chances are of being around when it's found.

These are some experiences of people with HIV or AIDS. Every body is different. People have to make up their own mind what's best for them.

Terry is in film production in Van Nuys, California.

"Although my last CD-4 T-cell count had jumped from 443 to 657, the next was 515—still not bad, and that reading happened during a minor sinus infection. Now it's in the upper 500's which is considered to be a high count.

"I didn't go into this with the power of positive thinking. Sort of a doubting Thomas. When my T-cell count went up, I was stunned more than anything. I really couldn't attribute this to anything other than Kombucha."

Joe in Cheyenne, Wyoming tells his experience this way.

"I'm a male, 36 years old who is HIV+. For the months of Sept thru Nov 94 I had nausea which kept me from eating, resulting in a 35 lb weight loss. Although I had been receiving medication for the nausea it caused me to have diarrhea which also lasted well over two months.

"Since drinking the Kombucha tea the cramping and diarrhea has stopped and I have gained seven lbs in the last 30 days. My M.D. says that it is mostly likely the medications which are responsible for the improvements. But I *know* it's the tea."

Tom is an artist in Mesa, Arizona.

"I am living with AIDS. For the last four years I have been challenged with the most severe eosinophilic folliculitis, primarily on my arms and legs. Five dermatologists, 'boo-coo' bucks, no relief. I started Kombucha in mid November.

"Today, my arms are *totally* healed and the legs are coming along nicely. I'm so happy not to be covered with scabs and sores. It seems my mental health has also improved, a state of well being. My art has taken a playful attitude.

"This *is* a magical gift from God and I treasure my 'buchees.'

"Not only surviving with AIDS—but thriving with AIDS."

CANCER

Cancer is one of the leading causes of death in the United States—each year it claims over half a million lives. It takes many different forms and can strike at almost any age, though the likelihood of discovering cancer increases with age. As we've mentioned, Kombucha is not a cure for cancer. It may, however, have a role to play in cancer treatment.

The American Cancer Society (ACS) defines cancer as a group of diseases characterized by uncontrolled growth and spread of abnormal cells. If the spread is not controlled, it can result in death. Cancer is traditionally treated with surgery, radiation, chemotherapy, hormones and immunotherapy.

	Total	Men	Women
Respiratory system	162,950	99,470	63,480
Digestive organs	124,330	66,130	58,200
Genital organs	67,380	40,980	26,400
Leukemia, blood, lymph tissues	54,850	29,220	25,630
Breast	46,240	240	46,000
Urinary organs	22,900	14,600	8,300
Brain, central nervous system	13,300	7,300	6,000
Bone, connective tissue, skin	12,080	7,050	5,030
All other and unspecified	42,970	24,010	18,960
Total	**547,000**	**289,000**	**258,000**

Source: ACS Cancer Facts & Figures—1995

Deaths from Cancer in the U.S. (1995) Est.

The probability that a treatment will actually remove the cancer varies considerably, and the life expectancy of people with cancer who do or do not have treatment also covers a wide range. A treatment is normally considered a success if the person lives for five years after treatment. According to the ACS, about 40% of the people diagnosed with cancer today will still be alive in five years.

We do not recommend using Kombucha instead of traditional medicine's cancer treatments. But it may be valuable in combination with those treatments. Or when used as a companion with other alternative treatments. Consider the following.

Chemotherapy is one of the most common treatments for cancer. It consists of giving a person chemicals that selectively destroy cancerous tissue. The process is generally repeated several times, with recovery periods in between. And recovery is needed. Common symptoms include loss of hair, mouth sores, lowered blood cell count, weakness and vomiting.

For information on cancer:
American Cancer Society
1599 Clifton Road NE
Atlanta, GA 30329
(800) 227-2345

Many people dread the impact of the symptoms so much that they refuse chemotherapy. You should know, however, that Kombucha seems to help people recover from the effects of this treatment. Frequently we're told by people going through chemo that their blood cell count rebounds much faster when they drink the tea. Other side effects also seem to clear up faster.

With bone marrow transplants, the stakes go even higher. This is still regarded by many doctors as an experimental procedure. As far as we know, it is only used if needed after traditional chemo. The treatment is more extreme. The number of people who have had the treatment and survived for five years is apparently not high, though we could find no definite numbers.

The bone marrow process consists of removing a small amount of marrow from the patient's pelvic bone, then administering such a powerful dose of chemotherapy that it kills virtually every blood-producing cell in the body. After the high dose chemo, the person's bone marrow is put back in and their body begins to produce blood cells again. It's not something done lightly. Side effects, in addition to extremely low blood cell count, can include having one's skin turn orange, loss of hair, loss of skin from hands and other areas, sores and secondary infections.

Lois, a lawyer in Atlanta, Georgia describes her experience this way.

"I have received a bone marrow transplant because of Stage III breast cancer. I had no mouth sores or infections and was taken off all antibiotics. My doctors were baffled because of my body's resiliency and how I was able to function after [this] near death experience."

Some people with cancer who do not have to go through chemotherapy or bone marrow transplants use Kombucha also. This is one of those experiences. Eric is a property developer in Beverly Hills.

"I have now been drinking…Kombucha tea for several months. I have prostate cancer and am a patient of an oncologist…. I am on a combined hormone treatment and also have…tea three times daily. I told [my doctor] and he seemed quite interested and said, 'By all means—go ahead with drinking this tea.' I do believe it is beneficial.

"I also have a hiatus hernia [which] causes me severe pain at times. Previously I found that a good tot of whiskey relieves the pain. But now I find that Kombucha tea can also stop this pain and obviously I now turn to this instead of relying on alcohol.

"I start off every day with a small glass of Kombucha tea, without any sugar or anything, and I find it a great way to start the day."

CHRONIC FATIGUE

People who come down with this devastating disease frequently find themselves unable to hold a job, and sometimes even bed-ridden. If that wasn't bad enough, more than one person told us their doctor ran some tests, couldn't identify anything, and told them it was all in their head. There is no known cause or cure for this disease.

The full name for this condition is chronic fatigue and immune dysfunction syndrome (CFIDS). The short form is chronic fatigue syndrome (CFS). The primary symptom is severe loss of energy to the point of not being able to do physical activity for more than a short period of time. Other symptoms may include short term memory loss, muscle pain, multi-joint pain and unrefreshing sleep.

According to the CFIDS Association of America, this is an illness that affects many different body systems. Fortunately, it is not necessarily a permanent condition. Since there is no cure, doctors frequently prescribe medicines for individual symptoms and suggest bed rest until it goes away—which may take months or years.

Now if there was just something that helps all parts of your body get back to normal…. Kombucha? Maybe.

For information on chronic fatigue:
CFIDS Association of America
P.O. Box 220398
Charlotte, NC 28222
(800) 442-3437

Two people who have CFS talked to us under condition that we not use their name. Apparently some employers place a stigma on people who have—or once had—chronic fatigue, as though "they just aren't willing to work." Strange.

The situation is made more difficult by people confusing it with other disorders, including multiple sclerosis, fibromyalgia and Epstein-Barr virus (EBV).

Fibromyalgia involves pain in the muscles, ligaments and tendons. The problem is only identified as fibromyalgia if it has lasted at least three months and involves at least 11 of 18 specific "tender points." The Fibromyalgia Network [P.O. Box 31750, Tucson, AZ 85751. (520) 290-5508] reports that roughly 75% of CFS-diagnosed patients will meet the fibromyalgia criteria.

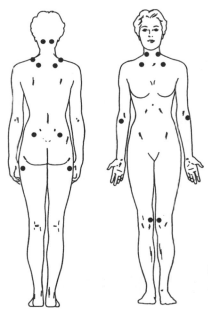

Source: *Fibromyalgia,*
Arthritis Foundation.

Fibromyalgia Tender Points

Most people with chronic fatigue try not to get bogged down in all the details. They're not doing well physically, want to get better, and the medical community seems to have little to offer in terms of handling this condition. Not surprisingly, many people with CFS turn to alternative treatments.

Kombucha is only one of a number of things people with chronic fatigue have used. Apparently the tea has often made big improvements, but is not a cure. A combination of treatments may prove to be the answer, but more information is needed. Here is what some people have told us.

A woman in California reported that after 7 months of being virtually bed ridden, she started drinking Kombucha and 2 days later was up and vacuuming the house!

Trudy in Ohio told us her experience.

"I suffered from this debilitating illness for some 8 or more years. If you know anything about this illness, you'll know there is no known cause or cure as of yet. I virtually lost my life, friends and myself. Until last October, I thought the nightmare would never end. [My sister received a mushroom, made the tea and] let me try it in Oct. of 1994. After 2 weeks, I felt that my illness was virtually gone.

"I have a whole different outlook on life now. I feel that God saved me...and gave me a second chance in life.... Not so long ago, I lived on pills and injections from my doctor just to survive. I wanted to just die and get it over with so I wouldn't suffer any more. Now, I know I can get up in the morning and feel good. It's great.... I have a new job, and I'm accomplishing things I never thought possible."

INDIGESTION, ULCERS, STRESS

Kombucha tea is slightly acidic, so people with indigestion or ulcers often assume they can't drink it. Not true.

It turns out that indigestion and stomach upset are often caused by incomplete digestion of food, though it may also be caused by ulcers. Properly prepared Kombucha tea has roughly the same acidity as your stomach. Drinking the tea adds to the digestive fluids produced by the stomach and seems to return things to normal—and even help the digestive cycle move forward so that "problem food" goes away.

Many people with sensitive stomachs report Kombucha helps them get through meals more comfortably.

For example, Mary Ann of Tucson, Arizona says, "I can't believe how great the tea is. I have had a stomach malady for 20 years. [After] 3 days of Kombucha (thanks to my neighbor) I am feeling better already. And what an appetite...yeah!"

Ulcers are believed by different people to be caused by different things. Some people feel ulcers are caused by on-going indigestion which eats away at the stomach lining. Others believe it is caused by stress—a domineering boss or a dangerous environment.

Lately, a bacteria called *Helicobacter pylori* (in short form, *H. pylori*) has been labeled the villain.

It is unlikely that any of those is the cause, all by itself. Strong evidence points to *H. pylori*. But this little bacteria is a normal part of our environment. Problems only occur when it starts going hog-wild and eating into the stomach lining, creating an ulcer.

Stress could easily cause the wrong amount of digestive juices to be present in the stomach, throwing off the normal balance and allowing *H. pylori* to take root and multiply. Similarly, repeated indigestion could cause local "hot spots" of undigested food to ferment, giving rise to conditions that let the bacteria multiply.

How does Kombucha enter into all this? We've already talked about the tea helping to advance the digestive process, which lets the stomach get back to normal. And under normal conditions, *H. pylori* does not seem to get out of control.

But there's more. We've also described how Kombucha appears to help all parts of your body work the way they're supposed to. When that happens, people frequently say they feel more "at peace." Some people talk in reverent tones about feeling closer to God. People express it in different ways—but almost everyone mentions it.

A person who is more "at peace" is less likely to suffer from stress. And a person whose body is working in a normal manner is less likely to suffer the chemical imbalances that seem to go with stress.

Anne in Hollis, New York says, "For some reason I was having headaches when I started taking [the] beverage. Headaches left immediately. I am very heavy. I lost 18 lbs.

"I had a lot of stress. Sometimes I felt like just collapsing. I no longer have stress. I am able to do more."

Pauline in Grand Junction, Michigan adds, "A friend helped me start on the tea three months ago. I had suffered from severe indigestion for at least 25 years. After six weeks on the tea I was able to forget about the tums and soda, etc."

MIGRAINE, ARTHRITIS, RHEUMATISM

These three physical maladies involve intense pain. Migraine is an extremely severe headache, usually confined to one side of the head. Arthritis is the inflammation of a joint, often accompanied by pain and structural changes. Rheumatism is a disorder of the hands, feet or back which is characterized by pain and stiffness.

Kombucha is not known to contain specific anti-pain medicine, but many people with these physical problems say it helps them.

For example Dan in South Bend, Indiana reports, "I have been using Kombuchas for about 6 months now. I have had arthritis in my hands...for about 36 years. I am 42 now!

"I started noticing a relief from the arthritis, as well as a general feeling of well being after about a week. You get a lift from the tea as soon as you drink it the first time."

Consider why you feel pain in the first place. It's your body's early warning to your brain that something is not working right. If there's a cut on your finger, you feel pain. It's a message telling you to stop doing whatever caused the cut (such as carelessly using a knife) and to take care of the cut so it doesn't get infected. Pain is not an accidental thing. It's always for a reason.

When you're in stressful situations, adrenaline can make your heart pound rapidly and constrict your blood vessels. This can cause a huge pressure rise in your blood vessels and make you feel pain.

According to the National Headache Foundation, migraine headaches are characterized by severe pain and, in many cases, nausea, vomiting, dizziness, cold hands, shaking, and sensitivity to light or sound. Attacks can last for several minutes or several days. 16-18 million Americans suffer from migraines annually.

> *For information on migraine and headaches:*
> National Headache Foundation
> 428 W. St. James Place, 2nd Floor
> Chicago IL 60614
> (800) 843-2256

The Arthritis Foundation describes arthritis as a general term that refers to more than 100 rheumatic diseases. It affects the body's joints—and warning signs are pain, swelling, stiffness or difficulty moving one or more joints. Nearly 40 million people in the U.S. have arthritis.

Normal joints have soft cartilage to cushion the bones, and the joint is enclosed in a capsule called the synovium. The synovium's lining releases a slippery fluid that helps the joint move smoothly and easily.

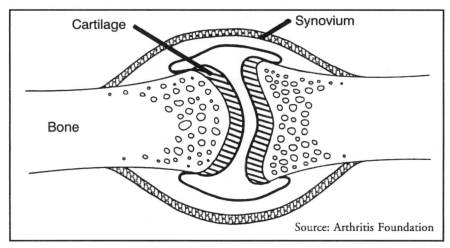

Source: Arthritis Foundation

Normal Joint

Joints with arthritis usually have inflammation and swelling. If the inflammation persists, it can damage the joint structures, including destroying part of the cartilage.

For information on arthritis and rheumatism:
Arthritis Foundation
1314 Spring Street, N.W.
Atlanta, GA 30309
(800) 283-7800

You can take a painkiller for migraine, arthritis or rheumatism, but what does that cure?

In a sense, taking a painkiller is backwards acknowledgment of holistic medicine. The painkiller doesn't cure anything. But it does give you a few hours without pain—during which time your body might heal itself. If not, a few hours later you take another painkiller, then another.

Kombucha will not stop a sudden pain. It doesn't contain highly concentrated chemicals like you find in prescription and non-prescription pills and capsules. Kombucha is a gentle treatment that seems to work over time to relieve causes of pain.

With arthritis, Kombucha may help to reduce the inflammation. Also, when your body is working correctly, producing the right hormones and nutrients in the right balance, some of the damage might be improved, or at least not get worse.

In our opinion, good health doesn't come from letting pain happen and then treating it. Health comes from keeping your body working right so pain doesn't happen.

Here are more experiences of people dealing with pain.

From Barbara Hallberg who owns a busy day care center. "Before taking [Kombucha] I was on a walker with arthritis in my knees. I am now running. No walker. No pain. I was in such pain before...I could hardly survive. What a miracle. No pills, no shots, no cortisone!"

Marsha in North Hollywood, California adds, "I have crippling arthritis and my fingers were starting to curl inward. After about three months on the tea my hands straightened out. I don't mean to say that the arthritis is cured. It's just that I can use my hands in a normal way."

Finally, Gayle in Atlanta Georgia shares this experience.

"I have a post-surgical arthritic condition in both knees. Having had knee surgery over 20 years ago, my knees were in such bad condition that I have friends who have never seen me walk without a limp until now.

"I wish I had the vocabulary to communicate my joy in reporting that I no longer limp. The day I discovered that I had gotten out of bed that morning and could walk to the bathroom, I cried. Chronic pain is so exhausting and debilitating.

"Chronic limping also attracts unwanted attention. Previously, I had to stop going to shopping centers because my legs simply would not support me on an expedition through the stores. There were times that I could not go to the grocery store or hardware store because, even with a handicap sticker, I could not get out of my car, walk to the store, shop, go through the checkout lane, return to my car and get home without excruciating pain and often, tears. The experience may be one that other people share occasionally, but for me, this was a nearly everyday event.

"I have torn up my handicap sticker for my car."

SORE THROAT, COLDS, FLU, ALLERGY, ASTHMA

This is a group of related disorders which, unlike the diseases described in other sections, happen to just about everybody. They are also "general health" issues, because if you keep yourself healthier, you are less likely to have problems with them.

Their symptoms are closely related, and sometimes it's hard to tell them apart: coughing, runny nose, watery eyes, breathing problems and sneezing.

A "sore throat" pretty much describes its problem. A "cold" is a breathing disorder characterized by sneezing, sore throat and coughing, caused by an allergic reaction or by a viral or bacterial infection. The "flu" is short for influenza, which is caused by viruses and characterized by breathing problems, weakness, exhaustion and inflammation of breathing passages. An "allergy" is a reaction to pollen, dust, medicine, etc., and often indicated by a runny nose, itchy eyes, wheezing, skin rash or diarrhea. "Asthma" is a breathing disorder, often allergic, characterized by lung spasms, wheezing, difficulty in breathing, and sometimes coughing.

There are two basic approaches to dealing with these problems. Some people take a series of medicines like cough suppressants, decongestants, pain relievers, etc. If the problem gets serious, they go to a doctor and get prescriptions for stronger stuff.

Other people rely on folk remedies like chicken soup, green tea, honey, garlic, etc. In fact, the Wilen sisters—Joan and Lydia—have gathered dozens of familiar and unfamiliar family cures into a popular book called *Chicken Soup & Other Folk Remedies*. They show several cures for any problem you can imagine.

Kombucha is different than either of these two courses of treatment because it's not something you take to cure a specific problem, like a hacking cough. Usually, after you come down with heavy symptoms, you're not going to get "instant relief" with the tea. At best, you might notice some symptoms going down after two or three days. For heavy symptoms, you may as well bring on the heavy-duty medications to attack the specific problem.

One of the most commonly reported effects of drinking the tea is general health improvement—and help in avoiding colds and other problems in the first place.

An exception to this rule is a sore throat caused by something other than a virus. For example, a personal experience by Sandy. "When I'm with friends who smoke, it sometimes gives me a scratchy, burning feeling in my throat. Drinking a little Kombucha makes it go away in a few minutes."

Rita Coolidge, who makes her living with her voice, says, "I have to drink the tea every day because it helps my throat when I'm singing a lot. I also find it helps with jet lag. I don't feel tired and have lots of staying power energy."

Among the people who drink Kombucha and have experiences with colds, allergies, asthma and similar problems is Joyce in Heber Springs, Arkansas. "My allergies are 90% gone—my asthma, gone. I don't have hot flashes any more. I have healthy fingernails [for] the first time in my life. And my gray hair is turning back to its natural color."

Maureen of Albuquerque, New Mexico reports, "I had been drinking the tea for five months when I went on vacation for two weeks. I didn't take my tea with me to drink and before I knew it I was sick with a cold. The first five months previous, I was never sick. I felt good and had lots of ambition.

"I will never go without my tea again. A friend of mine made a batch for me before I got home so I could start taking it again right away."

OTHER AILMENTS

People have reported a variety of other health improvements with Kombucha. We do not have enough information to comment on all of them, and some observations cover a range of areas. This is a sampling of those experiences.

HERNIA

Jim in Los Angeles, California.

"I have been suffering the pain of a hiatus hernia for about 15 years and was getting worse as the years went by. I have been drinking the Kombucha tea for two months. I have not had any pain since. I can eat anything I feel like, and I haven't been able to do that for many years. Prior to my knowledge of [the] tea, I was considering surgery."

HEMORRHOIDS/PAIN

Anne, a former nurse in Hollis, New York.

"My blood pressure dropped. I had not been able to sit up in bed without grabbing the mattress and pull & push until I could sit up, with terrible pain. Now I can sit up with no trouble. I have back damage from an accident and arthritis. I dragged my left leg when I arise in the morning. Now I can pick it up.

"Hemorrhoids were very painful before I started taking beverage. The pain subsided immediately. I've had no pain since."

EYES

Thom in Munith, Michigan.

"My parents are drinking their share [of tea] and they both reported eye sight problems. It turns out that their eye sight is improving rapidly, and their glasses aren't working as well as they were!"

BLOOD CLOTS

James, retired airline pilot in Irving, Texas.

"My wonderful M.D. recommended Kombucha because I have trouble with blood clots. Kombucha has heparin.*

"Actually, I learned about it first from a Franciscan priest in the Philippines. He said it kept him healthy. He gave me a mushroom about ten years ago."

BLADDER

Jane, a molecular biologist in Chicago, Illinois.

"I have been brewing my batches for a month now....

"I have recurrent interstitial cystitis. Since drinking Kombucha tea, my cystitis has calmed down to almost nothing! I read an article re: cystitis (the interstitial kind) in which heparin was used as part of the treatment and helped allay symptoms (pain, frequent need to urinate). I found it quite interesting that one component of Kombucha tea is heparin!* I had been drinking cranberry juice or tea, and although it helped, the Kombucha tea seems to have done the trick! I have since taken to brewing the Kombucha tea (using green tea) and mixed it (after brewing) with brewed cranberry tea to which I also add raspberry tea bags: 3-4 cranberry tea bags and 2 raspberry. This makes an excellent and delicious drink. My boyfriend loves it!

"It's going to be a lifetime drink for me."

[*An important clarification: Kombucha tea does not actually contain heparin. It contains glucuronic acid which your body can use—if needed—to make heparin.]

GULF WAR SYNDROME

Rosalie of Burbank, California.

"[My cousin] is suffering from Gulf War Syndrome. He has problems walking, severe pain in his joints, a respiratory problem and lack of energy.

"Since he has been drinking the tea he looks and walks just like he used to when we were kids. He is not a believer in holistic medicine but his energy level has come back to a point of his being unable to ignore the good results."

GENERAL EXPERIENCES

Karen is a herbologist in Milwaukee, Wisconsin.

"I am up to 10 mushrooms now and very excited about the results.

"My friend with MS has improved 75% since taking it. From bed ridden to day time driving—she's come a long way.

"I've had a slow, steady weight loss. Hurrah!

"My 96 [year old] grandmother overcame pneumonia in just days."

Sally Ann is a bookseller in Culver City, California.

"My tea mushrooms are getting bigger and look wonderful to me. The beverage itself has softened my skin and made it shine. My fingernails are stronger, my caffeine addiction has been transformed into enjoyment, not need. My appetite seems to be getting fine-tuned and I have an increased desire to drink pure, clean water.

"I am just beginning to consume 12 ounces per day (tea beverage), so it will be interesting to see what the future produces for me in combo with the Kombucha. I do notice obviously a sense of gentleness and well being."

SENIORS' PROBLEMS

Seniors do not necessarily have different problems than those described in the previous sections. The difference is usually in the sheer number of problems—some small, some large—and the impact they have on a person's life.

Remember the basic principle we mentioned earlier...we're born in excellent shape (most of us) and problems build up slowly over the years. It's not surprising that people who have survived enough of life's ups and downs to earn the title "senior" may have accumulated a number of physical problems.

The American Association of Retired Persons (AARP) reports this progression of ailments and years.

Age:	45 to 64	65 to 74	75+
Arthritis	253.8	437.3	554.5
Hypertension	229.1	383.8	375.6
Hearing Impairment	127.7	239.4	360.3
Heart Disease	118.9	231.6	353.0
Cataracts	16.1	107.4	234.3
Deformity or Ortho-pedic Impairment	155.5	141.4	177.0
Chronic Sinusitis	173.5	151.8	155.8
Visual Impairment	45.1	69.3	101.7
Varicose Veins	57.8	72.6	86.6
Diabetes	58.2	89.7	85.7

(Number per 1,000 people in 1989)

Source: *Aging America, Trends and Projections*, prepared by the U.S. Senate Special Committee on Aging, the AARP, the Federal Council on the Aging, and the U.S. Administration on Aging, 1991, Washington, D.C., p. 113. Primary source: National Center for Health Statistics, "Current estimates from the National Health Interview Survey, 1989," *Vital and Health Statistics*, Series 10, No. 176, October 1990.

Ailments and Years

How does Kombucha figure into this? The U.S. Department of Health studied Kombucha drinkers in an average American town in 1995. They mentioned that prior studies had indicated seniors in the U.S. do not normally use alternative medical treatments. But they found Kombucha to be the exception.

Why do large numbers of people over 50 turn to Kombucha? The answer, many of them tell us, is that it works.

The reference that comes up more often than any other when talking with seniors is the movie "Cocoon." Most people remember this story of older folks who discover a miracle bath that restores much of their youthful vigor and physical ability.

The results people describe after drinking the tea are amazing. And we don't mean just physically. The renewed sense of energy and enthusiasm seems to open new doors. The tremendous knowledge and experience they've accumulated over many years are being freed from physical limitations that held them back.

We believe those talents will soon be flowing back into the community at a greater rate than before, as people find they have the energy and health to do it.

> *For information on aging:*
> American Association of Retired Persons
> 601 E Street, N.W.
> Washington, D.C. 20049
> (202) 434-2277

There are a number of spirited personal stories by older Americans included in other sections of this book. Here is one more.

Anna lives in Boca Raton, Florida.

"A Russian man, who works with my grandson claims that they make this tea in Russia and then they also eat the mushroom.

"I don't know if it is mind over matter BUT I sure feel good since I'm drinking this tea drink. I feel so much stronger and my energy is coming back. I'm using this tea for approx. 4 months— I now walk 1½ to 4 miles two and three times a week—don't feel dizzy any more. I'm 77 years young (every little bit helps). However, I am not on any medication—I hate to take medicine—don't want to fill my body with anything but food if possible."

SAFETY

Since Kombucha is so new to the United States there has been some concern over whether it is safe. It's best to err on the side of safety and check it out. When you do, you'll see there are some things you should be concerned about—but you may be surprised at how safe it is when you make it correctly.

Some dreadful statements have been made by a few people that have no basis in fact. We'll look at the good, the bad and the ugly, and try to answer your questions.

CONTAMINATION

Is it possible for Kombucha to become contaminated?
Yes. Any food can be contaminated when not handled properly.

If Kombucha is prepared correctly, is it likely to become contaminated?
No. The danger associated with Kombucha doesn't come from the tea. It comes from people not preparing it correctly.

Is it difficult to make Kombucha the right way? If it's too difficult, maybe I shouldn't be doing it.
No. Actually it's easy to make it correctly. Just follow the steps in this book. People have been making it right for 2,000 years. It's not difficult. Betsy has made over 10,000 Kombucha mushrooms. None of them has ever been contaminated.

HOW BAD IS THE DANGER
IF IT REALLY GETS LOUSED UP?

In most cases, not bad. But there can be exceptions.

Early in 1995 a woman died in Iowa. People thought it might have something to do with Kombucha. The U.S. Department of Health investigated. Their study showed Kombucha was not found to be the cause (see the Rumors section).

In fact, in it's 2,000 year history, no one has ever been known to become seriously ill or die from drinking Kombucha tea. Compare that to the number of people who die each year from reaction to traditional medicines like aspirin or penicillin.

If someone messes up the Kombucha-making process, there's usually a clear signal. They look into the bowl when it's time to harvest the tea...and see mold.

In those cases, a person's health is perfectly OK if they do the logical thing—throw the mushroom and tea away. Then get a fresh mushroom from a friend and start over. But they should do it *right* next time. Find out which step was done incorrectly and fix it. When it's done right they won't have this problem.

Some problems have nothing to do with mold. If a person makes the tea in plastic, ceramic or another container which violates the instructions, small amounts of bad chemicals can get inside you when you drink the tea.

How do we know this? Betsy started her career as an industrial designer for a major manufacturer of food containers. Using the wrong container can cause a serious risk of chemical leaching.

Reactions in these cases usually amount to a skin rash, insomnia or other low-grade difficulties. But the long-range damage could be much worse. For most of the centuries of Kombucha's existence, users were protected by lack of technology. They had no plastic, lead crystal, etc. Certainly not in village huts. So prolonged use of plastic bowls or glazes containing cobalt, etc., have not been studied. Please. Follow the directions.

The danger of mixing Kombucha with traditional medicines? No negative reactions seen so far. In fact, some people say it helps their other medications work better and do what they were supposed to do. We recommend the safe course—tell your health care provider that you're drinking Kombucha tea.

WHAT DOES THE U.S. FOOD AND DRUG ADMINISTRATION (FDA) HAVE TO SAY ABOUT ALL THIS?

There's one key point on safety that many people seem to overlook. If the FDA thought Kombucha wasn't safe, they'd have taken it off the market. In fact, the FDA has checked Kombucha carefully, and even visited Betsy personally to check out Laurel Farms' growing methods. In a turnabout of normal roles, she lectured them about the importance of making it correctly and using proper containers to avoid contamination. She gave them Kombucha mushrooms to grow so they could see for themselves.

The FDA performed many laboratory tests on the Kombuchas and the tea they made, and issued a summary of their findings in a Talk Paper on March 23, 1995. They said, "The product contains considerable quantities of acids commonly found in some foods such as vinegar, and smaller quantities of ethyl alcohol. Because the acid could leach harmful quantities of lead and other toxic elements from certain types of containers—some ceramic and painted containers and lead crystal—such containers should not be used for storing Kombucha tea.

"The unconventional nature of the process used to make Kombucha tea has led to questions as to whether the product could become contaminated with potentially harmful microorganisms, such as the mold Aspergillus. Such contamination could produce serious adverse effects in immune-compromised individuals.

"FDA studies have found no evidence of contamination in Kombucha products fermented under sterile conditions. FDA and state of California inspections of the facilities of a major Kombucha tea supplier [Betsy's Laurel Farms] also found that its product was being manufactured under sanitary conditions.

"However, the agency still has concerns that home-brewed versions of this tea manufactured under non-sterile conditions may be prone to microbiological contamination. FDA will continue to monitor the situation...."

We have found the FDA to be thorough and reasonable in their investigations. We stand by their findings.

WHAT CAUSES THE DANGERS MENTIONED ABOVE?

The only known source of danger in Kombucha is carelessness in the person making the tea. The tea itself has remarkable protections against contamination, as we'll see later.

But if someone doesn't care if it's made right, it *is* possible to mess it up. These are the known sources of danger with Kombucha:

Why do I have to wash the bowl? It's just tea.

Believe it or not, some people don't clean the utensils they use to make Kombucha. We don't mean sterilize. That's going overboard. (Though we talked to a man with AIDS who sterilized everything. In his position, we might too. By the way, he was doing better, last we heard.) No, it just means wash everything with soap and hot water, and rinse well. Follow the other cleanliness steps mentioned in the "How to Make Kombucha Tea" chapter. It's mostly common sense.

Why buy a glass bowl? I've got this great plastic one.

As we describe in the "How To" chapter, using the wrong utensils can cause petroleum by-products, lead and other toxic materials to be leached into the tea. If you use a clear glass bowl and the other proper utensils, no problem.

Why just one recipe? I've got these great herbal teas I've been dying to try.

Kombucha depends on live, healthy bacteria and yeast to make the tea. Changing the recipe changes the tea. In some cases (as explained later) it can kill the healthy bacteria and ruin the Kombucha. Besides making the tea weaker or useless, it also lowers the tea's defenses against contamination.

Don't get us wrong. Herbal tea and other natural products are great. You can drink them in the same glass as Kombucha tea. But please don't use them to grow the tea. Someone with a serious ailment might get one of your baby mushrooms—and they may need to get the full benefit.

Why tell my doctor I'm drinking Kombucha? He or she will just laugh at me like when I tried garlic.

Don't worry about that. You're the one who pays the bill—the doctor works for you. You want their best advice. And you want them to listen to what you have to say. It's your health, and it's important.

If we have one concern that really stands out, it's that Kombucha might start getting your body back to normal—and you keep taking heavy doses of traditional medicine anyway.

Some people swear Kombucha helps traditional medications work better. That sounds good. But it's possible to get too much medicine. For example, too much insulin can be as dangerous as too little. Don't keep this a secret from your doctor.

PROTECTION AGAINST CONTAMINATION

Pop quiz. Which is likely to become contaminated first:

The milk in your refrigerator, or Kombucha tea?

Answer: *The milk.*

The hamburger you get at the coffee shop or Kombucha?

Answer: *The hamburger.*

The coffee sitting beside you at work, or Kombucha?

Answer: *The coffee.*

It's true. Prove it for yourself. Leave them out on the kitchen counter for two days. They'll be curdled, rancid or have mold growing on top. Except for the Kombucha tea.

Here's why it's true.

Kombucha has several natural levels of protection from outside contaminants. Some foods might have one of them. We haven't found anything else that has all of these.

ORGANIC ACIDS

Since before recorded history began, people have been preserving food by pickling it in organic acids. Kombucha has a wealth of organic acids. Two of them in particular—acetic acid and lactic acid—are widely recognized as excellent protection against the unwanted microorganisms that often try to get a foothold in everyday food.

The combined effect of all the organic acids in the tea causes it to be slightly acidic as soon as it's made, then it gradually becomes more acidic as it "grows." This level of acidity (pH = 3.5 to 2.0) makes it very difficult for any unhealthy bacteria to grow in the tea.

Samuel Page, in the FDA Natural Products Division, compares growing Kombucha to making pickles. He points out that you can leave pickles floating for months in a mold-ridden basement and not worry about contamination. But leave a cup of coffee out for a couple of days and you get household mold growing on it. He adds, "as the [Kombucha] culture is growing, it does become quite acidic, which is beneficial and would inhibit the growth of other organisms."

ALCOHOL

The fully-grown tea that you drink has very little alcohol in it. But during the early part of the "growing" process more of it is produced, and gradually converted into the organic acids described above.

Alcohol, even in small amounts, is excellent protection against mold. In wine-making it is well known that grapes bring mold spores with them from the field. But as soon as the grapes are squashed and fermentation begins, the first, small amounts of alcohol are enough to wipe out the mold.

CARBON DIOXIDE

The small bubbles that you often see in Kombucha tea are carbon dioxide—the same bubbles that occur in carbonated soft drinks. Carbon dioxide is a widely-used preservative. It's very effective against many microbes that try to grow in food.

ANTI-BACTERIAL EFFECT

Many studies of Kombucha have reported that the fully-grown tea has a mild anti-bacterial effect which protects it against other bacteria. These include Russian studies by Sakaryan and Danielova in 1948 and Barbancik in 1958, as well as a study in the United States by Hesseltine in 1965.

This effect is sometimes attributed to the presence of usnic acid and sometimes attributed to the organic acids in the tea.

RUMORS

When something is "new" there's very little factual information available, so incorrect information starts to travel. They're known as rumors. Kombucha is no exception.

The only cure for rumors is to provide actual information, in black and white, so people can check out the facts. Once that's done, rumors tend to evaporate.

That's why we did the research needed to produce this book. So you can check out the facts. Some of the most obvious rumors are dealt with here. Others may pop up later, but with any luck this data will handle them too.

MOROCCO

Kombucha has been widely used in Asia and Europe for a long time, and one way or another it got to Northern Africa. It became immensely popular, especially among poor people who couldn't afford Western medicines. Then a rumor started: drinking the tea will cause a mushroom to grow inside your body and take over your soul! Overnight, thousands upon thousands of Kombucha mushrooms were thrown into the streets.

Come on. Unless your insides are made out of tea and sugar, there's no chance a Kombucha is going to grow. When you eat bean sprouts on your salad, you don't get beans growing in your stomach. Even when people eat the mushroom itself, and some do, it's rapidly digested.

But in Morocco the general level of ignorance on this subject was high, and the rumor was enough to rob them of the benefit they had been getting.

IOWA

In a small town in Iowa, like in many parts of America, one person got a Kombucha mushroom, enjoyed what happened for them, and gave baby mushrooms to their neighbors. Then their neighbors did the same. In April, 1995, two women became ill and one of them died. No immediate cause was found. So a rumor started: Kombucha will kill you!

The media picked it up and played it across the country. Some people became scared and stopped using Kombucha.

The U.S. Department of Health had been carefully monitoring Kombucha through the FDA, as we have seen. To be on the safe side, the Department commissioned an extensive study into what happened in Iowa. The Centers for Disease Control and Prevention (CDC) was given the lead role, with the FDA and Iowa Department of Public Health actively participating.

They contacted people in the town and found over a hundred were drinking the tea, with no ill effect. Hospital records were examined—it was very thorough.

For eight months rumors circulated while the study continued. On December 8, 1995, the CDC reported the results:

1. "Samples of the mushrooms and samples of the tea consumed by both case-patients were sent to FDA for analysis.

2. "No known human pathogens or toxin-producing organisms were identified.

3. "The investigation described in this report did not establish a causal link between the illness of the two women and their consumption of Kombucha tea."

Unfortunately, media stories about the final report were confusing, even though the report was clear.

See for yourself. To get a copy of the report, write to Centers for Disease Control and Prevention, Atlanta, GA 30333 and ask for a copy of "MMWR Vol. 44, No. 48."

After extensive testing by the country's top health agencies, the clear result is that no causal link was found to Kombucha tea.

NO GLUCURONIC ACID?

Glucuronic acid is one of the key organic ingredients found in Kombucha tea. As discussed in the "History and Research" chapter, it helps the liver detoxify your body. All laboratory analysis of Kombucha over the past hundred years has shown it to be present. Then in 1995 a new rumor started: there's no glucuronic acid in Kombucha tea!

The otherwise well-respected person who made that claim published his results and gave the name of the lab that did the work.

Shocked, to say the least, we called the lab.

Their response? They're not equipped to test for glucuronic acid. We checked the published report. They told the truth. For several substances the report said "negative." It did not say "negative" for glucuronic acid—it was not on the list!

The researcher simply made an assumption.

That's how rumors start.

Dr. Philippe Blanc, of France's National Institute of Applied Sciences, recently confirmed glucuronic acid is present in Kombucha tea.

DIABETES

The basic ingredients for making Kombucha tea are well known: sugar, tea, water and Kombucha. Sometimes people stop there and go ballistic. "Sugar! A person with diabetes can't drink that!"

People who bother to find out the whole story know that isn't true. The sugar is mostly used up during the 7 to 10 day "growing" process. For a more detailed discussion, see the "Diabetes" section.

HIV/AIDS

A similar thing happens with HIV and AIDS. By now every-one knows Kombucha is a combination of bacteria and yeast. Some people stop there and take off. "Yeast! A person with HIV/AIDS can't drink that!"

Again, people who bother to learn the whole story know that's not true. This is not the dangerous spore fungus, it's healthy budding yeast (see the "Yeast Infection" section). And the tea is not an antibiotic which could trigger an auto-immune disease (see the "Antibiotic?" section).

You'll notice several experiences in this book are told by people who have HIV or AIDS. They drink the tea and have had good results.

Oddly enough, it's mostly people who *don't* have HIV/AIDS who complain about Kombucha's "risk." People with HIV or AIDS are highly motivated to do their homework. And when they've done it, they often start drinking the tea.

MUSHROOM PEOPLE

Individuals who study mushrooms are called mycologists. They're experts in real mushrooms—like toadstools. Not Kombucha.

You've heard it enough times by now that you know Kombucha is not a mushroom. It's a bacteria-yeast combination. People call it "mushroom" because it looks like one.

Calling your sweetheart "honey" does not mean they were made by a bee on a summer afternoon. It's just an expression.

That little "mushroom" misunderstanding has resulted in some very strange behavior. Some mycologists who sell real mushrooms are opposed to Kombucha. We mean red-faced, sputteringly op-posed. In fact, the most irresponsible claims made about Kombucha have been made by mycologists who sell real mushrooms.

Two of those claims are: It's an antibiotic, and antibiotics are dangerous! It's moldy!

The several people who have said this always start by making one of these statements: "I don't know about Kombucha, but I think...." or "I have made Kombucha so poorly it's been covered with mold, so I think...."

Those are not particularly good credentials. Now if a mycologist were to say, "I've grown many of them successfully, and I think...." *that* would be worth hearing. We've talked to some very intelligent mycologists. Surely some of them will be getting up to speed soon.

ANTIBIOTIC?

High on the rumor list: Kombucha is an antibiotic! Using it will make other antibiotics not work! People will get auto-immune diseases!

Amazing. First of all, if antibiotics are such a threat to the world's survival, perhaps doctors should stop giving them out. But that's beside the point. Because Kombucha is not an antibiotic.

Many studies have reported Kombucha has a mild anti-bacterial effect. Much like vinegar. This was documented not only by European studies, but by Clifford Hesseltine, president of the Mycological Society of America. They were precise in their reports and did not identify Kombucha as an antibiotic. They refer only to gentle antibacterial effect.

If you have strep throat and go to a doctor, don't let him prescribe Kombucha tea. It won't be much good for that. Get an antibiotic if you want a cure from him.

Auto-immune disease occurs when an organism that is commonly found in a person's body starts growing rapidly, gets out of control and causes symptoms. Real antibiotics target specific illnesses, but may have the side effect of weakening your body's natural defenses and allowing auto-immune diseases to occur.

As we've seen, Kombucha is not an antibiotic. It works to build up the body's natural defenses.

MOLDY?

Another top hit on the rumor list: Kombucha is moldy! It's a danger to people with compromised immune systems!

As you saw in the Safety section, mold does not grow on properly prepared Kombucha. None of Betsy's 10,000 mushrooms had mold. Chances are, that's more mushrooms than the average person will make. Even the FDA showed no contamination occurs when it's done right.

A person has to do something wrong to get mold. That doesn't mean they're a bad person at all. It just means they missed some step—like leaving the tea out overnight to cool, or preparing it beside some nice, attractive flowering plants. When they figure out what's wrong, they don't get mold.

We've noticed that people with HIV or AIDS are very careful to make the tea correctly. They need the benefit. They can't afford problems. None of them has ever told us they saw mold.

As we've explained, Kombucha has many built-in protections against mold of any kind. It's one of the last things in your kitchen that's going to get mold. It's remarkably safe.

IT CURES EVERYTHING!

Good grief. Talk about exaggeration. The two places you're most likely to see this rumor are on some of the anonymous instruction sheets that people type for making the tea, and in the media.

It makes for good hype, but not for good health.

If other people want to say that stuff, OK. For us, and we hope for you, it makes more sense to be realistic.

Kombucha seems to do a lot of wonderful things for people. But we've said it before and here it is again. Kombucha is not a cure for anything. Your body cures itself. Kombucha just seems to help your body do that.

We hope that by the time you've considered all the different aspects of Kombucha we explore here, you'll have an appreciation for how remarkable your body is, and how Kombucha can play a significant role in your health.

DO'S AND DON'TS	
DO	**DON'T**
Clean your hands and the work area before you start.	Have houseplants near the tea.
Use black or green tea.	Use herbal or Earl Grey tea.
Use distilled water.	Use chlorinated water.
	Use an aluminum pot to boil the water.
Use refined, white sugar.	Use brown sugar or honey.
Use a clear glass bowl.	Use plastic, crystal, ceramic or colored glass bowl.
Cover with a clean, white cloth.	Cover with cheesecloth or plastic wrap.
Hold the cloth in place with a rubber band.	Leave air gaps around the cloth.
Make new tea right away when old tea is harvested.	Let Kombucha mushroom sit in the open air before making tea.
Use a clear glass container to store the tea.	Use a plastic, crystal, ceramic or colored glass container to store the tea.

HOW TO MAKE KOMBUCHA TEA

It's easy to make Kombucha tea the right way, once you know how. And it's *important* to make it right. As we explained Kombucha has natural protections that keep it healthy—and help you keep healthy. But if you make it wrong, and unfortunately there are many incorrect instructions out there, it can lose its protections and cause unwanted side effects.

We described to you how the FDA checked on Kombucha to see if it was safe for public use, and visited Betsy. She emphasized to them the importance of doing it *right*. She gave them a Kombucha mushroom and a copy of her instructions then sent them on their way.

Later, the FDA issued their Talk Paper which found no evidence of contamination in Kombucha when made properly. But they expressed concerns about what might happen if people don't grow the tea correctly.

If you decide to get a mushroom and make Kombucha tea, there are a few clear, easy steps you should follow.

People refer to this as the Betsy Pryor Method, but so far as we know, this is the only way to make the purest, most effective tea. It was created after searching through information and records that came from Europe and Asia where the tea has been made for many generations.

Some people like to experiment with variations on this method, or say that certain precautions in handling the mushroom and tea are not necessary. For all we know, damaged mushrooms and weak tea may still produce some benefit. But to tell the truth, it hurts to even consider it.

Please. Start by doing it right. Completely right, as shown in the following pages. Get the full effect of Kombucha tea. After you see the results, we think you'll always want to do it this way.

BEFORE YOUR MUSHROOM ARRIVES

Once you've arranged to get a baby Kombucha from a friend or grower (see References chapter) you'll need to get a few things ready. It's like preparing for the arrival of another kind of baby. You're better off getting things ready before the event. (Good news: no diapers!)

HERE'S WHAT YOU'LL NEED

A 3- OR 4-QUART GLASS MIXING BOWL. The larger bowl is better to hold the full batch of tea you're going to make. The smaller

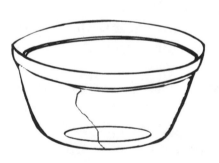

bowl will work, but it's a very tight fit. Use clear, uncolored glass only. *No plastic, ceramic or crystal!* Later we'll explain how the tea may help to detoxify your body. For now, all you need to know is that it will try to detoxify the bowl. It'll pull out things like lead from crystal, cobalt from ceramics and petroleum by-products from plastic—and leave it in the tea. Who wants to drink that stuff? Plus it can get into the mushroom and stay for a long, long time. Use clear glass only! (Pyrex, Anchor-Hocking, Libby or Luminarc is good). Don't use a jar. Your Kombucha mushroom needs a large air surface for breathing space.

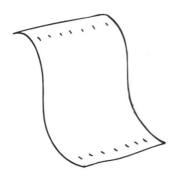

A WHITE BAKING TOWEL, FLOUR SACK CLOTH, or anything made of white, pure cotton and breathable. An old, white, clean T-shirt, cut into a square will do. In fact, it helps to have two of them so you can use one while the other's in the laundry. No cheesecloth, ever. It's much too porous

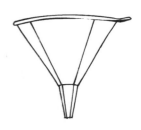

and little fruit flies could get through. When you're ready to harvest your health beverage in a week or so, you can use the white cloth to strain the tea as you pour it through a **FUNNEL** into your refrigerator container. Then you can toss the old cloth in the wash and continue with the clean one.

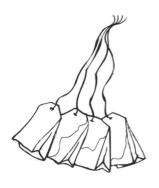

FOUR TEA BAGS of black tea (Lipton orange pekoe cut black tea is okay). You can use three bags of green tea and one of black, if you prefer. (Some people believe green tea has anti-cancer properties.) Don't worry about the caffeine. There's almost none left at the end of the fermentation process. We'll talk about herbal teas later—they react in some good and not-so-good ways with the Kombucha. But while you're getting started, please stay with black or green tea.

A LARGE, SIX-INCH RUBBER BAND. A piece of string *might*
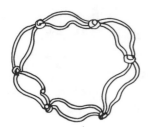
do. But we don't think you can get the tight fit with a string that keeps fruit or vinegar flies from crawling under the white cotton cloth. If you don't have one, large rubber band, try tying several smaller ones end-to-end and make a circle big enough to stretch around the bowl.

A WOODEN OR PLASTIC SPOON. No metal should touch your mushroom! It tarnishes metal quickly, and that rusty stuff can get in the mushroom and tea.
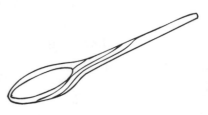
Ugh! Don't do it. Remember to remove rings and jewelry from your hands before touching the mushroom. They're metal, right? (If you can't get a ring off, wear plastic gloves.)

ONE CUP PURE WHITE CANE OR BEET SUGAR. Okay,
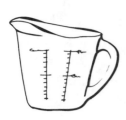
okay. The stuff probably isn't healthy. Well, the mushroom eats it, not you, so just grit your teeth and pour. Besides, after a week to ten days, the sparkling health beverage you'll harvest has almost none of this sugar left.

Why not brown sugar? Russian scientists studying Kombucha found refined white sugar produced the best results. Brown sugar contains molasses and the mushroom can't digest it. Never use honey—it can kill or cripple the key bacteria in the Kombucha.

STAINLESS STEEL POT OR PAN, MINIMUM FOUR-QUART SIZE. We've used up to twenty-four-quart restaurant-quality stainless stock pots. (Bigger pots are great if you're making more than one batch of Kombucha.) You can use a metal pot because it won't come anywhere near the mushroom. But no aluminum! They get tarnished just sitting around in the kitchen. By the time you're ready to make tea, the stuff rubs off. Not good.

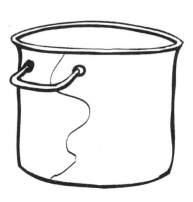

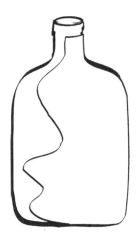

CLEAN, CLEAR WATER—3 quarts or more. If you're lucky enough to have pure well water where you live, no problem. The rest of us need to stop by the store and pick up some distilled water or use a water purifier. Just make sure there's no chlorine or other gunk in the water. And no water softeners.

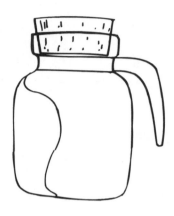

GLASS REFRIGERATOR CONTAINER to store the tea after your first "harvest." Each mushroom will produce about one or two quarts of tea, so plan ahead and get one or more containers. Clear glass only, and it's best if the container has a lid. Plastic lids are okay as long as they don't poke down into the tea.

That's what you need. If you have these things on hand before the Kombucha arrives, you're all set to go!

SUBSTITUTIONS?

One rule. No ingredient or utensil substitutions. Ever. No matter what. Over the years, Kombucha has thrived where care was taken. It's also died out where not properly handled.

If you substitute honey, artificial sweetener or something else for sugar, or use herbal or decaf tea instead of black or green (the essential oils in some herbal or fruited tea can kill the mushroom), the healthy properties of the Kombucha tea are destroyed, and you might as well drink a soda pop.

Yes, yes, you say. The "babies" grown with substitute ingredients can look pretty good. But they're only ordinary yeast patties now, not true Kombucha.

THE FIRST TIME YOU MAKE TEA

You probably received your mushroom in an airtight plastic bag from a friend or distributor. Open the bag and let the mushroom

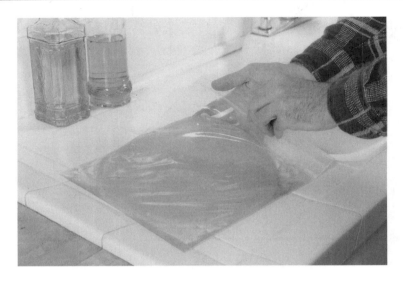

New mushroom arrives

breathe. Whew! It's going to smell "vinegary" but that's okay. Make sure you don't spill the tea inside, because you'll need it to "start" the fermenting process.

To keep your mushroom happy and healthy, don't let it come into contact with metal, direct sunlight or microwaves. Those things may cause it to break out in spots or even die. Much better to give it a little tender, loving care.

SO LET'S COOK!

Start by cleaning your hands, utensils, bowls and kitchen counter. Make sure dishes are out of the sink and there are no houseplants, fruit or open food containers around. The Kombucha has great defenses against mold spores and unfriendly bacteria, but don't take chances. Keep things clean!

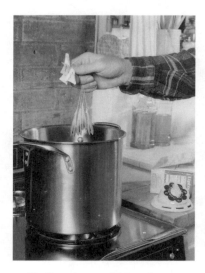

Boil water, add tea bags

Bring 3 quarts of water to a boil (remember, distilled is best) in your stainless steel pot. Add 1 cup sugar and boil for another five minutes.

Turn off the heat, add four tea bags and let them steep for ten minutes. Remove the tea bags and let the brew cool a bit.

Ladle or pour the tea into your see-through glass mixing bowl. Let the tea cool to room temperature. Hot tea can damage the mushroom, so make sure it's cooled.

Add 4-6 ounces of the old tea at this point (if this is your first time, pour it from the plastic bag your mushroom came in.) Then gently place your Kombucha mushroom on top of the "growing tea." Let the darker, rougher side of the mushroom float face down in the new tea.

If needed, put two pieces of tape or something similar (no metal) across the top of the bowl...this keeps the white cloth from dipping into the tea. Cover with the cloth. Tie with string or pull the rubber band around the cloth to secure tea and mushroom against fruit flies, mold spores, etc. Place bowl in dim or dark, quiet,

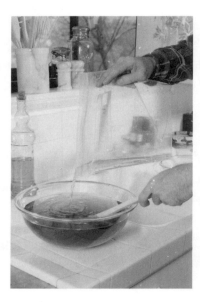

When new tea is cool, add old tea

84

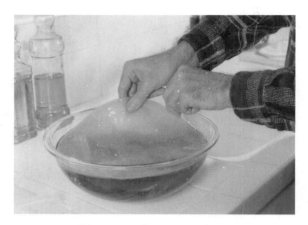

Place mushroom on tea

temperate, clean spot (about 70 to 90° F) with adequate air-flow—such as a shelf in the kitchen, cellar, open closet, loft or attic. Not on the floor, if possible.

Remember, direct sunlight can kill your mushroom, so be careful. Also, the mushroom will give off a mild, vinegary smell, so keep this in mind when choosing its new home. Don't move it around after the initial placement—that disturbs the fermenting process.

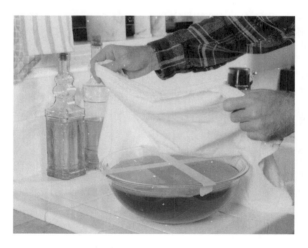

Cover with cloth

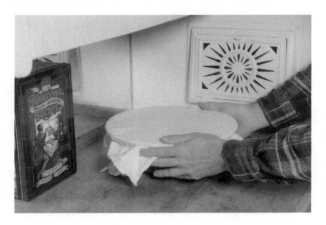

Put bowl in dim, quiet place

AFTER SEVEN TO TEN DAYS...

You're ready to harvest your new baby mushroom and refrigerate your sparkling health beverage! Remove the white cloth from your glass bowl. Notice that the "mother" mushroom (the one on bottom—the original one) has given birth to a baby (the one on top). Make sure your hands are clean and take off any jewelry (no metal, remember?). Remove both mushrooms from the bowl (they might be stuck together) and separate baby from mother by pulling apart gently.

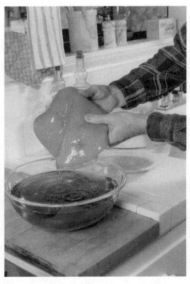

Remove mushrooms from bowl

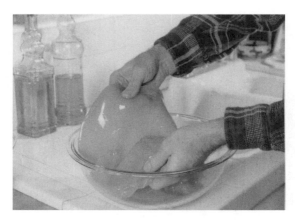

Separate baby from mother

Put them in another glass bowl or deep dish with just enough newly harvested tea to cover them.

Now pour the newly fermented Kombucha tea from the glass bowl (using the white cloth as a strainer) into a clear glass container (the funnel is a big help here) and place your tea in the refrigerator. All right! Chill, and it's ready to drink.

We'll tell you more about storing and using the tea later.

NOW, START AGAIN RIGHT AWAY

Don't let mushrooms sit on the counter for more than 30 minutes. Leaving them out longer can

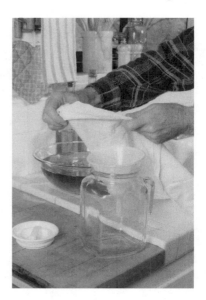

Prepare to pour tea...with funnel and white cloth

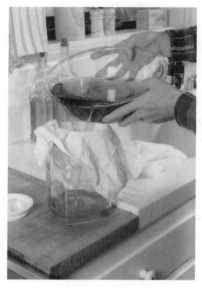

Pour through the cloth

attract mold or fruit flies and weaken the culture. And *never* put them in plastic bags to store in the refrigerator. This can cause toxic reactions and cripple the mushroom.

Brew a fresh batch of "growing tea" using the two mushrooms. You can double the amount of tea you make by putting each mushroom in a separate bowl. Just double the recipe (water, tea, sugar) and follow the same steps.

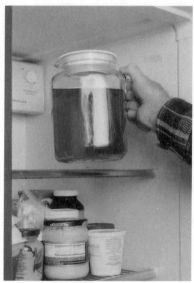

Store tea in refrigerator

HOW MANY MUSHROOMS WILL YOU WANT TO KEEP?

That depends. We've discovered that after seven to ten days of fermenting, the 3 quarts of liquid you made will yield about 1¾ quarts of Kombucha tea. If you drink the recommended 12 ounces a day (that's 84 ounces a week or about 2½ quarts) you'd need to ferment two mushrooms per person to make enough for 7–10 days. In Eastern Europe and

Asia, families grow their mushrooms in larger bowls. You can do this, too. Simply adjust the recipe to reflect the number of quarts in the larger bowl.

Always remember that the mushroom needs a large surface to "breathe." So no "sun tea" jars, small-mouthed containers or fish bowls. Don't worry if the larger surface area is bigger than your mushroom. When you make the first batch of tea, the mother will make a baby mushroom that exactly fits the new, larger container!

PROBLEMS THAT MAY COME UP AND WHAT TO DO ABOUT THEM

BUBBLES

The Kombucha mushroom is kind of ugly in a cute sort of way. Don't worry if it gets little bubbles or "warts." These are usually on the side that faces down in the "growing tea," and are simply air pockets. Gently press the bubble out with your hands.

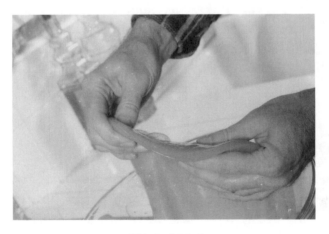

"Air bubble"

HOLES

The side that faces up is usually shiny, smooth, and lighter in color, but not always perfect. If holes form when you separate the mom from the baby, don't worry. Your Kombucha will still make a terrific tea.

MOLD

If for some reason you get mold on your mushroom (we've never seen this, but people say it happens) older sources say to just remove it by dunking the mushroom in a bowl of vinegar for a few minutes, then rinsing under the tap. But...we recommend starting with a fresh mushroom and not drinking or using that tea as "starter." Some molds have no effect. Others could be very harmful.

To avoid getting mold in the first place, follow the easy instructions in this book. Normally, you won't ever get mold unless something isn't done right. That's because the Kombucha tea is slightly acidic, and eliminates most germs that come near it. It also has mild anti-bacterial ingredients that give added protection.

Kombucha tea is protected better than most of the food in your kitchen. How can you help the Kombucha protect itself? Don't leave the mushroom exposed to air for a long time during "harvest." Always add 4-6 ounces of old tea to the new batch. Don't put your Kombucha near any plants. Keep it covered with a cloth while it's growing. Keep the tea in a covered container in the refrigerator after harvest.

SHRED

If the mushroom looks a little "worse for wear" after harvesting, rinse it under the tap in lukewarm water (unless you have heavily chlorinated water—then dip in distilled water or use a water purifier). This will clear off the harmless, little brown culture "tags."

TOO HOT

Putting the mushroom into new tea that is too hot (over 100° F) can cripple or kill it. Always let new tea cool to room temperature before adding the mushroom or the 4–6 ounces of old tea.

If your mushroom drops to the bottom of the bowl, it can mean the tea has not cooled enough. Unless the tea was *very* hot, your mushroom is still okay. Don't worry about it.

WORN

If the mushroom turns really brown, it might be old and tired. Discard (bury it in a garden or whatever) and continue with the baby. If treated with love and kindness, the offspring of your mushroom should last a lifetime.

CROWDED

You shouldn't put more than one mushroom into a batch of tea. Believe it or not, some people don't remove the babies, and let the mushroom get very, very thick. This will cause some of the mushrooms to starve—there's not enough nutrients in a batch of tea for all of them. Use one mushroom in each bowl of tea, and give the others away.

THIN

If your baby mushroom is thin and scrawny when you harvest it, that usually means it was too cold. Try to keep the temperature between 70 to 90° F. In winter, it may help if you put more than 4–6 ounces of harvested tea into the bowl of new tea before adding the mushroom—this helps jump-start the process. If the temperature falls below 70 degrees while it's brewing, give the mushroom two or three more days to grow. If it was not too cold, maybe something is vibrating near it, like a refrigerator, microwave, washing machine or car. By the way, they don't seem to do well with cigarette smoke around them.

VACATION

If you need to leave the mushroom alone for a month or two, float it in a 3–4 quart or larger clear glass bowl of "growing tea," covered with white cotton cloth and a rubber band. Place it in a cool, dim spot—your refrigerator will do—at about 42 to 48° F. When you return, throw out the old tea and make a fresh batch the normal way. Then start the harvest cycle again. It should be fine.

FREEZING

Never freeze your Kombucha. That only works in an industrial, quick-freeze unit. In a slow-freeze refrigerator (like you have at home) crystallization of water in the cells can occur, causing them to burst and cripple or kill the mushroom. If you're not going to use the Kombucha for a long time, give it to a friend or neighbor. They'll return the favor some day.

REPLACEMENT

That brings up something very important. Lots of times you hear people talking about using extraordinary methods to repair a Kombucha when it's been damaged. They try to cut out a piece of mold, or "breed out" contaminants caused by growing it in plastic. Don't do it.

One of the great things about Kombucha is that when you make a batch of tea, you get a free baby mushroom. You can use the first few mushrooms yourself, but will soon find you're up to your whatever in extra mushrooms. Give them to relatives, friends or people down the street. Let them share some of the good feelings you get from staying healthy.

And, let those people be your back-up in case your mushroom gets scalded or you go on a long vacation. You'll find they're more than happy to give you their next "baby"—clean, fresh and healthy.

HOW TO GIVE SOMEONE A KOMBUCHA

Once people experience the good health and good feelings that come with Kombucha, they often get excited about sharing it with other people. The great part is…you get a free mushroom after every harvest. You *can* share it—with friends, people at work or people you meet at social events. Here's how.

First and most important, raise your mushroom well. Keep your own Kombucha mushroom well-cared-for and it will produce beautiful babies.

If you tell people about your Kombucha experiences and they ask for a mushroom, agree to let them have your next "baby" (some people actually have a waiting list of relatives and neighbors). Don't stack your extra mushrooms in the refrigerator or freeze them like

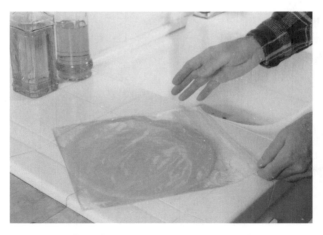

Give baby mushroom a friend

fish fillets—it can severely damage them. At the very least, it will reduce their ability to make beneficial tea for a while, and the person receiving your gift will probably assume (correctly) something is wrong. Give them a good experience. Give them only a fresh mushroom, directly from your harvest.

While they're waiting a few days for the fresh mushroom, you should advise them to get ready. They'll need to pick up things like a clear glass bowl, tea, sugar, and the other items listed in this book. To help, you should copy a set of instructions for them so they know what to expect and what to do. If you really care about them, you could give a copy of this book—or send them down to the bookstore to get their own.

When harvest day comes, you should have a plastic, freezer-quality, zip-top bag on hand. When you separate the baby mushroom from the mother, place the new mushroom in the bag and add 4–6 ounces of newly harvested tea. Then press the side of the bag gently to remove most of the air from it, and seal the top tightly.

Place the bag out of the sunlight and not near a microwave. It would be great, of course, if the person receiving the mushroom was standing right there and could run home with it to start their own tea. That rarely happens. But it should get into their hands as soon as possible, and they should get the mushroom into it's own bowl of tea within a few days—seven days at the most.

The fun part comes a couple of weeks later—when they've had time to make some tea and drink it for a while. You know that time has come when you see the smile on their face. The hard part is…then you have to listen to *their* great experiences. Oh, well.

HERBAL TEA

The good news about herbal tea is that it can give a different (some people say "much better") taste to the Kombucha tea. Herbal teas may also add beneficial vitamins and other good things.

The bad news is that using herbal tea to grow Kombucha may damage the Kombucha and drastically weaken the benefits of the tea. This happens because many herbs contain what is called volatile oil, and a high dose of it is harmful to the healthy bacteria in Kombucha.

Several references show the amount of these volatile oils in herbs, and that can guide you if you're serious about finding a way to include herbs in your Kombucha tea. Unfortunately, different references give different answers. Some recommend chamomile, others say "never!"

We recommend you brew healthy, herbal tea by itself and enjoy it—but not use herbal tea to *make* Kombucha.

Also…some people ask if they can heat Kombucha like other teas before drinking it. Don't! Kombucha tea contains organic substances that can be destroyed by heat.

WHEN YOU GET A NEW MUSHROOM

Is it healthy and well-grown? How do you know?

Without resorting to a lab analysis, it's really hard to tell. But there are some simple precautions you can take.

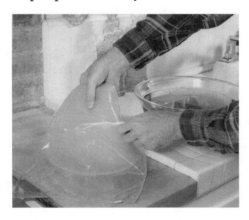

Check new mushroom carefully

Look at it to see if there is any mold. Politely ask the person giving it to you how it was raised. Did they use clean and careful methods like the ones described here? How long has it been out of its bowl of tea, sitting in a plastic bag? Seven days is the longest it can go before beginning to starve.

Be aware—a damaged mushroom will not give you good tea. And if it's moldy it can be dangerous. Be safe. Use a healthy mushroom.

MAKE A FRIEND

No time to raise a Kombucha while you race around in your hectic life? Is your house or apartment too small to give the Kombucha bowls their own growing space?

Find a friend in the neighborhood to make the tea for you. There's almost always someone in the neighborhood who's retired, a homemaker, or has a disability that keeps them close to home. Work out a trade. They may need help with a chore around the house or some other compensation. In return, they can give you a ready supply of Kombucha tea.

Actually, once a person is making tea for themselves, there's very little work in filling a few additional bowls for neighbors. And there's a tremendous payback—people who receive the tea tend to be very grateful and in good spirits. It's a rewarding experience.

If you're the one receiving the tea, remember a little appreciation goes a long way.

SUMMARY

The next two pages contain an easy-to-read visual summary of the "Betsy Pryor Method." Use it in combination with the detailed discussions on the previous pages.

THE BETSY PRYOR METHOD

1. Wash hands

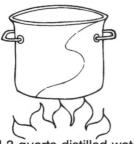

Boil 3 quarts distilled water

2. Add cup sugar

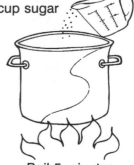

Boil 5 minutes

3. Turn off heat

Add 4 tea bags

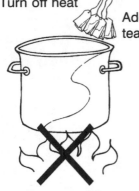

4. Steep tea bags for ten minutes

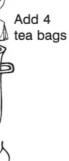

Remove tea bags

5. Cool tea to room temperature! Then pour into 3–4 quart, clear, glass bowl

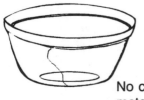

No crystal, metal, ceramic or plastic bowls!

6. Add about 4–6 oz. of newly-harvested tea

No suntea jars or cylinders, USE BOWL

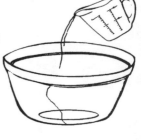

FOR KOMBUCHA TEA

7. Float mushroom on top of tea—rougher, darker side down

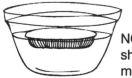

NO metal should touch mushroom

Room temperature

8. Put tape across top of bowl (optional)

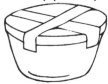

Cover with thin, freshly laundered white cloth, and rubberband

9.

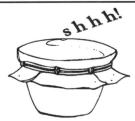

shhh!

Place in a dim, clean, quiet, ventilated space, 7–10 days, 70-90 degrees

10. Then remove mushrooms, gently separate

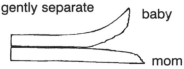

baby

mom

Start over right away. Don't store in plastic bags in refrigerator or leave out in open.

11.

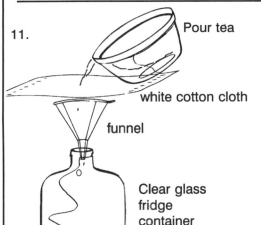

Pour tea

white cotton cloth

funnel

Clear glass fridge container

12.

People drink an average of 4 ounces three times a day—before, after or between meals. Whenever! To your health!

DRINKING THE TEA AND OTHER USES

The Kombucha health beverage tastes like a light Moselle wine or a really snappy apple cider. Normally, you drink 4 ounces on an empty stomach before breakfast. This gives you a terrific energy boost—a great way to start the day! Later drink another 4 ounces before lunch and before dinner if you want to lose weight. Or, if you're happy with your weight and want to help your digestive process, drink 4 ounces after lunch and dinner or any time in between.

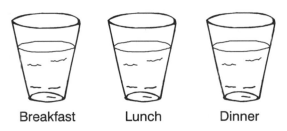

Breakfast   Lunch   Dinner

A real life experience: "Without changing my eating habits, I lost 14 pounds in a few months, and gained a wonderful feeling of renewed well-being and energy within the first week."

Everyone is built differently, but feeling better and having much more energy is described by many people.

Sometimes people drink more or less than 12 ounces a day. Let your body tell you.

Can you drink too much? Dr. Wydoff told us his Russian athletes drank up to 24 ounces per day. Ken in Berryville, Arkansas reported, "I have been drinking 2 qts a day with no side effects at all. Oh by the way I'm 6'3" and weigh 280 lbs and with the tea I have so much more energy I cleaned our whole house from top to bottom. This stuff is a Godsend!"

On the other hand, some people are perfectly satisfied with 6 ounces a day. Do what works for you.

If the refrigerated health beverage seems a little too strong for your taste, add an ounce of distilled water to your 4 ounce drink. Some people mix juices with the tea to give some variety to the taste, but it's possible that strong juices can interfere with the healthful qualities of the tea. If you really want a good, healthy result, only mix with water. If you're basically healthy and are just using this for a tune-up, go ahead and experiment.

But—never mix something with Kombucha tea and let it sit in the refrigerator or on the counter. The tea continues to "grow" slightly, even in the fridge. Putting something else in it can weaken the tea and possibly cause an unpleasant reaction. If you really want to use a mixture, do it in the glass just before you drink it.

Another way to adjust the tea to suit your taste is to make the fermenting time a little shorter or longer. A lot will depend on your climate, altitude, season of the year and even phase of the moon. Experiment. We've heard that brewing the tea for much less time (2 to 5 days) produces a sweeter taste but may reduce the benefits tremendously.

In winter it's colder and the tea doesn't grow as fast. As a result, it tastes sweeter. Let it grow a few days longer to get the same "summer" taste.

If you feel the tea is giving you some real health benefits and you want to get the most out of it, let the tea grow longer—ten to fourteen days. This makes the tea stronger, and also gives it a more tart flavor. It definitely packs a wallop.

DRINKING TEA THE FIRST TIME

Kombucha tea has its own natural flavor—which is reasonable considering it's extraordinary effect.

If you're a first-time drinker, or giving it to someone who is, there are a couple of things you should know.

The taste gets stronger as the tea grows. After 7 days it has a fairly mild taste. After 10, it's much stronger. Do first-time drinkers a favor: give them tea that's only grown for 7 days.

Also, the tea is always sweetest right after harvest. It tastes like carbonated apple cider. After that, the tea continues to grow slowly. By the end of the week, just before you make your next harvest, you'll notice the old tea tastes much stronger and a bit more "sharp."

Tip #2: give first-time drinkers newly harvested tea.

Some people compare Kombucha to drinking coffee. The first time most people try coffee, they wonder why it's so popular. After a while they find themselves at the local cafe paying extra to get the strong stuff.

When drinking Kombucha tea, quantity is also important. Don't overdo it at first. We recommend only drinking 2 ounces three times a day during the first week. By strange and wonderful coincidence, that's exactly how much tea is made by one mushroom.

After the first harvest, when you separate the baby mushroom from the mother, you can make two bowls of tea. That should produce enough for you to drink 4 ounces each time from then on.

STORING YOUR TEA

You'd be surprised. No matter how often it's mentioned, someone will store their tea in a plastic container. Please don't! As we pointed out before, the tea could draw out petroleum by-products, and you don't want to drink that!

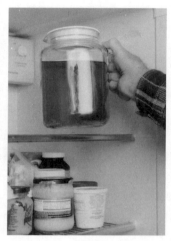

Store in glass container in refrigerator

Use clear glass containers only. And keep it refrigerated or cooled. You know by now that the tea continues to grow even after the mushroom is removed. Without refrigeration it may get sour before you have a chance to drink it.

If the tea has to sit out for some reason, shake it occasionally to keep a new mushroom from trying to form on top of it.

Even in the fridge, you'll notice some stuff settles to the bottom of the container. These are little bits of healthy yeast and shreds of mushroom. This is normal, and you'll tend to get more of it as the week goes on. Some people eat the little pieces of mushroom and swear

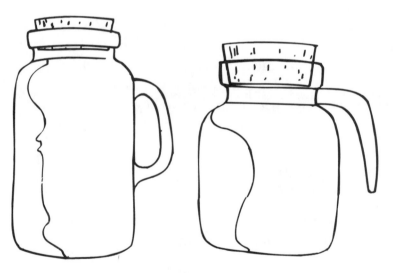

You can store the tea in any size bottle, but remember, the bottle must be clear glass

it improves their digestion. Some people leave it in the bottom of the jar and wash it out at the end of the week. It's up to you.

The tea shouldn't be kept in storage longer than a couple of months after it's been made. Old studies indicate that if Kombucha is bottled, it can keep for up to five months. But not when sitting in a container in your refrigerator. To be on the safe side, we recommend you feed the old tea to your plants and make a fresh batch.

Some enterprising people noticed that if the tea gets *very* old, it can taste like vinegar. So they actually use it for that purpose and sprinkle it over salads as a healthy substitute. Do whatever works for you.

KOMBUCHA TEA IN HEALTH FOOD STORES

Finding bottled Kombucha in stores is becoming more common now. It saves people the work of growing tea themselves. On the other hand, it's not cheap (about $5.00 per pint at places we visited) and the quality of the tea can vary widely.

We've never bottled it, since it's always available fresh. But we did talk to people at health food stores, bought some bottled tea and tried it. Here are some thoughts.

The cleanliness and care of the person making the tea are not apparent by looking at the bottle, so you should be careful to buy it from a reputable store. The benefit you get from the tea will also depend on how long it was grown. You have to hope for the normal seven to ten day period. Some producers might grow it for only two to three days so they can make more bottles of tea every week—good for them, but not so good for you. There could be little or no benefit from young tea. A short growing time and long "bottled" time might offset each other, or might not. Ask questions and use your judgment.

The taste of the beverage will change depending on how long it sits in the bottle, since it continues to ferment. An old bottle may taste somewhat sour.

Some bottlers also mix herbs, honey and other ingredients with the Kombucha. Check the label, and see if this is something you want.

If you decide to use store-bought Kombucha, reach for glass bottles only. No plastic.

SIDE EFFECTS?

So far the tea has been used for many generations, and when Kombucha is prepared correctly the only "side effect" mentioned is some nausea if a person drinks too much tea too quickly.

A doctor in Santa Monica had an experience with that. Several patients told him they use Kombucha, so he has had a chance to learn their experiences. One patient reported feeling nauseous so he recommended she stop for a few days. She did, then started again and felt fine.

Other side effects? Many studies have been done in Europe and Russia over the last hundred years (see References) and several times they said conclusively, "no side effects."

As mentioned in the Safety chapter, the FDA also ran tests on Kombucha and found no contamination when the tea is made correctly.

However, while speaking with people on our booksigning tour we found some individuals who said they had side effects. They reported rashes, insomnia and general aches. In every case, when asked how they were growing the tea, they were doing something wrong. Please—we want everyone to have a good experience with Kombucha. Do it right!

HOW DO YOU FEEL?

You should always feel the same or better after drinking Kombucha tea.

If something unusual happens and you feel worse, stop taking it while you check out the following possibilities.

Since the tea has a mild detoxifying effect, your body may need to adjust to the change. You might need to wait a couple of days, start with a smaller amount of tea, and gradually build it up.

If you're taking medications and drinking the tea, there is a possibility that might cause upset. We haven't heard reports of bad combinations, but play it safe. Consult your health care provider.

It's possible that you're fighting off an illness or flu that's going around. If you have symptoms, stop! Wait until the symptoms pass. Then you can try the tea again, with small amounts at first.

If one or more of the "clean and careful" handling methods for making and storing the tea have not been followed and the mushroom has become crippled or contaminated, you could have a physical reaction. If this happens, don't fool around. Throw away the mushroom and the tea made from it. Get a clean, healthy mushroom and start again.

And check every step. Somewhere along the line you'll find someone took a shortcut and put the mushroom in boiling tea, used a plastic container or something else. **No shortcuts.**

OTHER USES

Though the main use for Kombucha is as a healthy beverage, people have found other good ways to use the tea and the mushroom—as a facial tonic, for example. From a woman in Los Angeles: "I got the idea after the Northridge earthquake. After a week of living on a closed mountain road that looked like it had been hit by a bomb, my skin was a wreck! The stress of all the quake damage and after-shocks had aged it ten years. The Kombucha restored it to normalcy within a few days, and now my friends are telling me that my skin never looked better."

A couple Hollywood celebrities confide that they add a cup of Kombucha to their bath. Then while they're relaxing in the warm tub, they put a Kombucha on their face like a mask for 15 to 20 minutes. They swear this reduces pore size, removes fine lines and sunspots, adds healthy color and restores their skin to baby smooth-ness. An Australian grandmother even bathes with a dozen Kombuchas, claiming that this seems to energize her and relieve muscle soreness.

A Florida lifeguard reports that after a long day in the hot sun, nothing works better than a topical application of Kombucha tea to take the red out of a sunburned nose.

Directly applying a Kombucha mushroom to the burned area has apparently also helped. Jenny, a set painter in Hollywood, got a bad sunburn and put her mushroom on the worst area. The next morning, there was a tan circle where the Kombucha had been. The rest was still red and painful.

Pieces of Kombucha placed against skin rashes, herpes and cuts also seem to have a profoundly healing effect. A man working in his woodshop deeply sliced his index finger with an electric saw. Before leaving for the emergency room, his wife cut a piece of Kombucha and wrapped it around his bleeding finger. When they arrived at the emergency room, the physician checking the finger asked why the man had bothered to drive to the hospital through a raging thunderstorm with what appeared to be a paper cut.

People also report that Kombucha helps with nail fungus. Sim-ply drinking the tea seems to be enough to do it, though some people apply tea directly to the affected area.

Gargling with the tea has also been found to help with sore throat, bad breath, gum infections, plaque and tartar reduction.

Betsy can attest to this. At a recent check-up, her dentist was amazed that she had no plaque and asked what she was doing.

William, a hairdresser in Akron, Ohio, mixes the tea with water and uses it after shampooing as a finishing rinse. Other people report that this has eliminated dandruff.

Several school children used Kombucha in school projects, watering indoor and outdoor plants and vegetable gardens with a mixture of half water, half Kombucha tea. They noticed that it caused the plants to grow faster, flower more often, and develop leaves with a beautiful, healthy sheen.

A woman who buries extra pieces of Kombucha in her garden said that nearby bushes have twice as much new growth as the others in her yard. And some people living in snowy climates reported that their plants don't go through "winter slump" if watered occasionally with undiluted Kombucha tea.

A person who no longer serves alcohol at parties now creates a "snappy" punch with a mixture of 1/3 Kombucha and 2/3 fruit juice. And a bartender reported that a Kombucha "chaser" between drinks seems to counter the effects of alcohol, allowing people a safer trip home after a night on the town.

A number of people have mentioned that drinking a few ounces of Kombucha tea after meals takes away that "full" feeling and eliminates the need for antacids.

PET AND ANIMAL USES

Many people report benefits for pets and other animals similar to what people experience. Dogs and cats need only four to eight eyedroppers-full of tea in their water dish each day. Among aging dogs and cats the results are especially visible. These include improvements in their hair, hearing, eyesight and temperament.

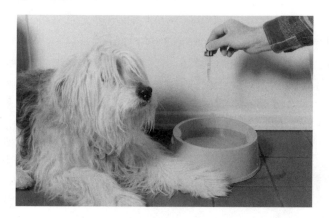

Four to eight drops can benefit your pets

During flea season, their skin can be soothed by mixing equal amounts of tea and water. Spray it on flea-irritated areas or apply it directly to the hot spot with a cotton ball.

For horses, up to a gallon of tea can be put into a standard trough filled with water. Farmers also report giving tea to ostriches, dairy cows and other animals, but we don't have information on how much tea was used.

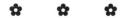

The following report on Kombucha treatment for animals was given to us by veterinarian Roger DeHaan, D.V.M.

As a holistic veterinarian with 28 years of medical experience, from the ivy halls of the university to 12 years in the jungles of South America, I am always looking for simple answers. I am intrigued by Kombucha tea, therefore, because it has a long history of use and research. And what could make more sense than conquering disease organisms with "good ones."

I approached Kombucha tea with my usual skepticism combined with an open mind. A valued client provided my first Kombucha "baby," with instructions. Intrigued, I researched the literature available—not wanting to be gullible—and armed with the facts I decided to try it on a few dozen pets. About a dozen of these were cancer cases.

Of course I did no double blind trials. All of the pets get diet changes and nutritional, herbal and homeopathic supplements, and some of them were on appropriate drugs. When improvement comes, and it usually does, I cannot attribute it to one "miracle pill or tea." Rather, I look for combinations that work, boost the immune system, and get the pet back into the fight for life. My experience is that Kombucha tea can be part of that combination, for many pets.

What I find is that the tea shows promise for many health benefits, with few negatives. The promise is that most pets need a healthier digestive system, and the ability to detoxify the chemical junk that is thrown at them in today's pet foods. The glucuronic acid, a key ingredient, seems to be part of the key, helping the liver to detoxify, regenerate, and do its 500 or so functions with flying colors.

As a holistic vet, I have seen hundreds of pets given up by the orthodox profession as being "hopeless." Of the ones I have treated holistically, and comprehensively, approximately 80% have responded positively. That gives me a lot of hope, so that I now tell owners that we can promise no guarantees, no exaggerated claims—yet if they are patient and want to try a nutritional and holistic approach—it is a path well worth following. Kombucha tea fits into this philosophy very nicely.

What really surprised me was that most pets like the tea—even some of the most finicky cats! I have owners add it to the food—or if their pets refuse to eat food, then dilute it with water, broth or some favorite food, and give it with a dropper or force-feed it. But most pets will eat it with relish!

Common sense requires that we start out with a minimum—a few drops or teaspoons as the size of the pet may dictate—then gradually increase it as the pet accepts the taste.

If a pet refuses the tea? Well, start with less—just a few drops. Never force the issue, however. I think pets are smarter than most humans. If they don't want it, in fact refuse the stuff, find a different road. Some animals are too "acid," and need to be alkalized first. The tea is not the place to start. They are trying to tell us something, and we must listen. But that does not mean it may not be good in a few weeks, or that some of the healthy pets might not be benefited "preventively."

If you drink the tea yourself, can I suggest you include your four-legged and even two-legged (bird) pets? Make it a family project! Although definitely not a "cure-all," there certainly are plenty of positive benefits!

I examined a poodle who was emaciated, poor appetite, depressed, rotten hair coat and rotten breath. We suspected but never proved cancer. He was not responding to other treatments. Within a few weeks, on a tablespoon of Kombucha twice daily, there was a definite turnaround, a whole new attitude to life. The haircoat and bad breath also improved dramatically. It was possible to get a doggie "kiss" again, rather than a face-full of halitosis. The owners were very pleased!

Another interesting thing is that Kombucha tea seems to enhance the effect of drug and natural treatments alike. Pets that are out of balance and nutritionally depleted seldom respond properly to any kind of therapy. Remember, even a drug is not a cure—it is the body that must cure. If the body is depleted, the drug becomes even more poison—more toxic. Get the body nourished, and it can deal with the drug—detoxifying its poisons, thus giving the drug a chance to work pharmaceutically. That is why I like the idea of prevention, keeping the pet well nourished and healthy. Then if drugs are needed, they have a better chance of being effective, with less harmful side-effects.

According to the U.S. Department of Agriculture (USDA) and the World Health Organization, our soils are 85% depleted of their natural minerals—because of our modern farming methods of raping the soils. If the soil which makes our food is depleted, so are our bodies. As a holistic veterinarian, I would encourage you to get serious about getting a variety of whole and balanced foods into your pet, with supplements. The "100% complete" dog food at the grocery store is neither complete nor is it healthy—or rather, it is guaranteed to keep your pet healthy for 26 weeks, then all bets are off.

So a better diet, with more variety, is a must. Then you may consider giving Kombucha tea as a regular supplement, to help the body assimilate the food with more efficiency.

*Dr. DeHaan is a graduate of Michigan State University and is the author of **Natural Care of Pets**, a book which contains more than 30 articles on pet health. To obtain a copy of the book, send $10.95 to Natural Care of Pets, RR1 Box 47A, Frazee, Minnesota 56544. He is also available for phone consultations at a reasonable fee for anyone wishing to inquire further about pet diet, supplements for prevention, or natural approaches to chronic diseases. For a phone appointment call (218) 846-9112, 9-noon Central Time on week days.*

HISTORY AND RESEARCH

CHINA

It is widely believed that as early as 220 BC in China—during the Tsin dynasty—people tried to find immortality through the use of fungus treatments, which they believed had magical properties. There was one variety prized above all others, known to the Chinese as Ling-tche, the Divine Tea. This is the unique combination of natural ingredients that has come down to us through the generations as Kombucha.

Today there is something marketed in China as "Ling-tche" which we are told is not Kombucha. If you happen to be shopping there, be careful.

Peggy in Seattle, Washington came in contact with the early roots of Kombucha through her husband.

"He is from Xian, which is the ancient capital of China…. He's been watching me doing this thing with the Kombucha and when he saw the first one I made, he recognized it immediately. And he said, 'Oh yes, my family made these mushrooms. And we drank the tea.'

"The first batch of tea I made was like nectar of the gods. And he and I both just consumed it right away.

"In China the whole entire family lives together…. He tells me this is something that went on in their family. This was a family project."

JAPAN

In 414 AD, the Japanese Emperor Inkyo was reported to be suffering from severe digestive troubles, and summoned a physician from Korea. This doctor Kombu is believed to have brought the divine tea to Japan.

Kombu is also the name of a Japanese brown seaweed, so watch what you get there.

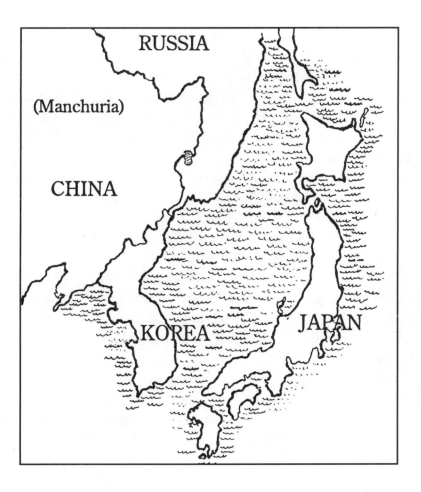

In later years, Japanese warriors considered the properties of this divine tea so special that they carried it into battle in their field flasks. This is believed to be one of the few times the tea was fermented on the move. Historical archives indicate that their habit was to top off the ferment in their hip flasks with fresh tea, allowing some of the old culture to ferment the new tea. They considered it a refreshing and strengthening beverage.

RUSSIA

Historians indicate that as trade routes extended, oriental merchants probably carried the mushroom with them to Russia. From there it made its way into Eastern Europe. The habit of drinking this fermented tea then became quite acceptable throughout Europe.

It is common to see stories of grandmothers tending a pot of Kombucha in the corner of small, rustic homes and doling it out to family members stricken by illnesses or other maladies.

One of the many local names given to Kombucha over the years grew out of this experience. A woman traveling in Russia saw that many villagers in Kargasok lived to ripe old ages in good health and she searched for their "secret." It turned out that each hut had one or more pots of this amazing tea brewing, and the tea was given to all members of the family as a normal part of their life. Reports of this miraculous "Kargasok tea" spread the use of Kombucha even farther.

Olya in Virginia tells her personal experience with Kombucha when she lived in Russia.

"I was born and raised in the former USSR, and I remember visiting my aunt and being treated to a very special sweet-and-sour tangy drink. I just loved it! My aunt kept a glass jar-bottle on her windowsill with a gauze covering the top, so 'it' could breathe but no dust or dirt would get in. We affectionately called it 'gribok'— little mushroom.

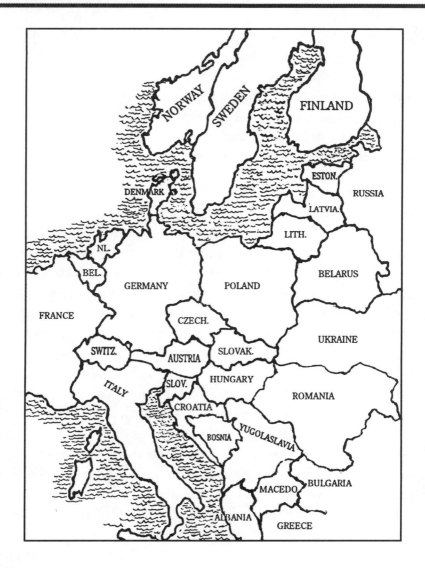

"Unfortunately, my mom thought it would be too much work for her to keep one 'gribok' at our house; so I had to wait for those infrequent visits to my aunt's.

"I've been in this country for 20 years now, and I always thought that 'gribok' was one of those things forever lost to me since I left Russia. So when I saw [Kombucha] it was like...coming home!"

EUROPE

As Kombucha was passed from family to family across Europe in the late 1800's, it attracted the interest of health professionals. German doctors and scientists studied the Kombucha mushroom and tea in great detail from 1900 until World War II. During the war, strict rationing and widespread shortage of two essential ingredients, tea and sugar, almost wiped out the use of Kombucha in Europe, including much of Russia.

Fortunately, some of the mushrooms were preserved and a resurgence of Kombucha began after the war. Italian high society, for example seemed to have had a real passion for this fermented tea during the 1950's.

As an interesting footnote, **Günther Frank** reports that in 1952 **Stalin's** personal physician (Vinogradov), aware of Stalin's fear of cancer, ordered tests on Kombucha, which was believed to help prevent it. Satisfied that Kombucha at least had no bad effects, the doctor gave this tea to the Soviet leader. Unfortunately, two KGB officers (Ryumin and Ignatiev) tried to improve their position with Stalin by claiming he was being poisoned. The doctor was jailed and rumors quickly spread that this drink (which Russians call "tea kvass") was likely to produce cancer. Use of the tea plummeted. When Stalin died in 1953, the KGB officers were put in jail and the doctor was vindicated. A book published in Russia by Barbancik in 1954 dispelled the rumor.

A few years later in the 1960's scientific research in Switzerland found that drinking Kombucha was at least as beneficial as eating yogurt. It's popularity soon increased and it became widely available again.

One of the people credited with extensive research into the properties and beneficial use of Kombucha is **Dr. Rudolf Sklenar** in Germany. He used it in his medical practice and gave the mushrooms to his patients from about 1951 until his death in 1987. He reported that "Kombucha produced good therapeutical results in cases of metabolic diseases, also with those of a chronical nature... In no instance undesired side or late effects caused by a treatment with these therapeutics were ascertainable." He recommended it as one of the beneficial treatments for people suffering from cancer.

Today, the two recognized authorities on Kombucha in Europe are Dr. Sklenar's niece and collaborator, **Rosina Fasching** in Austria, and Günther Frank in Germany.

UNITED STATES

The Kombucha mushroom has been in America at least since 1960, but was only used by a few individuals. People seemed to regard it as a private treasure and did not give them to "outsiders." The first crack in that private usage came in early 1993 when **Tom Valentine** published an article on Kombucha in "Search for Health" The next major breakthrough occurred in August of 1993 when **Betsy Pryor** obtained a mushroom and began her "Johnny Appleseed" crusade to get Kombucha into the hands of everyone in the country who wanted one.

Betsy got her Kombucha mushroom indirectly from Manchuria by way of Sister Joan Derry of the Brahma Kumaris Center. When Betsy gave baby mushrooms to her older neighbors, the quiet canyon street soon became active with people tending their gardens and showing more energy than they had in years. She gave other mushrooms to people in the AIDS community and saw similar effects. Based on those positive experiences, she began to distribute this productive strain of Kombucha across the country.

Over the past couple of years, she has grown and sent out more than 10,000 mushrooms, and each of them has been doubling every seven to ten days. Even if we assume two-thirds of all new mushrooms are discarded or used for something other than making tea, the descendants of her mushrooms probably number over two million in the United States today.

The Kombucha mushroom and tea are now available in all fifty states.

Prof. Eduard Stadelmann at the University of Minnesota has researched Kombucha for over fifty years. From 1957 to 1961, while teaching at Univerisität Freiburg in Switzerland, he published several widely-quoted articles which surveyed the field of research into Kombucha, and included over 200 references.

Stadelmann began using Kombucha in Europe in 1930, and is very familiar with the people who have studied it. In 1960 he sent a mushroom to **Clifford Hesseltine**, President of the Mycological Society of America, whose laboratory tests confirmed the tea produced antibacterial activity. The results were published in 1965.

Stadelmann keeps track of progress being made on Kombucha studies in Europe, and keeps in touch with people in the United States and around the world who work with it. He graciously provided us with copies of his work and excellent guidance in developing this book.

Dr. Jeffrey Gates and **Dr. Keith Steinkraus** at Cornell University are actively involved in the search for better understanding of the medical effects of Kombucha.

Dr. Steinkraus is a recognized expert in the field of fermentation, and has personally used Kombucha for eleven years.

Dr. Gates has worked with Kombucha for the past two years, and is particularly interested in it as a possible treatment for gastrointestinal disorders (ulcers, etc.) as well as examining its possible effect on tumors, cancer prevention, prostate and breast cancer. He reports that his "research done in cooperation with Dr. John Babish of Paracelsian, Inc., revealed that the Kombucha elixir does have a modest ability to inhibit tumor development."

We hope foundations and other institutions will provide the financial support to continue this good work.

Drs. Richard and **Rachael Heller** are very interested in Kombucha because it may be related to other work they have been doing. They are professors at Mount Sinai School of Medicine in New York, and the best-selling authors of *Healthy for Life.*

"A ROSE BY ANY OTHER NAME..."

As you might expect from something that has become established in many countries over hundreds of years, Kombucha is known by many names. These are some of the ones you may see when books or articles are translated into English from another language.

NAMES FOR THE MUSHROOM

Brinum-Ssene (Latvian)
Cainii grib (Russian)
Cainogo griba (Georgian)
Chamboucho (Romanian)
Champignon de longue vie (French)
Combucha (Japanese)
Fungus japonicus (Pharmaceutical name)
Funko cinese (Italian)
Hongo (Spanish)
Japán gomba (Hungarian)
Kargasok-Teepilz (German)
Kombucha (International usage)
Olinka (Bohemian and Moravian monasteries)
Tea mould (Java)
Teepilz (German)
Teyi saki (Armenian)
Theezwam Komboecha (Dutch)

NAMES FOR THE BEVERAGE

Cainii kvass (Russian)
  This is usually translated "tea kvass."
  Do not confuse it with "kvass," the
  Russian name for a sour beer.
Cainogo kvassa (Georgian)
Elixir de longue vie (French)
Kombucha tea (English)
Kombucha-thee (Dutch)
Kombuchagetränk (German)

Sometimes people talk about different parts of the Kombucha mushroom or tea, particularly in scientific studies. In those cases, you may see other names such as Saccharomyces (yeast), which we will explain as they come up

HOLISTIC HEALTH

The holistic view of health grew from ideas originally presented by **Jan Christian Smuts** in 1926.

He urged that medicine and science not be broken into small pieces and treated as isolated events. The interaction of different pieces is sometimes more important than what happens in any particular part.

This especially applies to chronic diseases. If the ailment is repeatedly treated with medicine but keeps coming back, the cause of the problem has not been found. A wider view is required.

Holistic health encourages that wider view. And encourages the use of a variety of methods which do not necessarily involve the use of drugs. Those methods tend to use stress reduction, removal of toxins, physical manipulation, natural herbs and proper diet.

The strength of holistic health is twofold: prevention of disease through proper care of yourself, and long-term health through helping the body to heal itself.

The strength of modern medicine is in handling high impact diseases and physical problems which require immediate response. Broken bones, ruptured blood vessels and high-fever infections are strong candidates for surgery or penicillin. The goal is to save a person's life.

There is no reason why the two cannot support each other. Mild, natural, long-term care may be the best way to prevent and treat many illnesses. But when paramedics in an ambulance pick you up at the scene of an accident and ask where you want to go, the hospital might be a very good choice.

A DENMARK EXPERIENCE

Lydia has a Ph.D. in chemistry from Carnegie-Mellon and has worked for biotech companies in Australia and the United States. But like most people, she didn't really know what "holistic" was. This is her story.

In 1984 I moved to Copenhagen, Denmark. It was a new country with a language I was trying desperately to understand. I was under a lot of strain at work—sometimes working 80 hour weeks.

I started to build up a small circle of friends, however the combination of language, work hours, new country and a much higher fat diet (my favorite lunch was lard sandwiches) started to take a toll. At this point in my life I knew absolutely nothing about my body, its functions and needs. I was a pure "head" person. My body was there to support my brain. I never put on weight so I did not think in terms of what I ate as making a difference or being something that I needed to consider.

Then I came tumbling down. I was on holiday on a once in a lifetime boat trip to the Arctic Circle along the Norwegian coast when I got a very bad flu. I was in my cabin—sick, very sick. It was an effort to go on deck. When the overland part of the trip started, I collapsed. Took the next train back and got antibiotics on the way home. They stopped my sore throat and fever. However I was so weak that I had to stay in bed for two weeks.

I went back to work on principle, not because I was better. I would sleep ten hours at night, crawl to work, come home and go back to bed. The weekends I spent in bed. I went to four different doctors. I did not have mono or worms or parasites—or anything wrong with me as far as they could tell. This was very discouraging news. Did it mean I was always going to live like this—that it was "normal?"

A friend at work recommended a naturopath. I had no idea what that was but I definitely needed to do something. I had been to enough doctors to get a consensus on what they could help me with at this point in time. So I broadened my horizons. It turned out to be a life changing decision. The naturopath was **Kurt Winberg-Nielsen.**

He did some tests (which I did not and still do not understand) which showed that my organ functions were very low. It never occurred to me to consider my organ functions. He gave me a prescription of vitamins, minerals and herbs to build up my system. I also learned that I was supposed to drink water, at least eight glasses a day.

Slowly but surely it started to work. In the meantime I had time to read his book on health and healing (in Danish so it was slow going—but then I had time). I think that his theory makes a lot of sense and have summarized a small part of it here.

Biopati—en vej til sundhed (Biopathy—a way to health)
by Kurt Winberg-Nielsen.
Narayana Press. Gylling, Denmark. 1982

What is sickness? Sickness is the situation which appears when the body is subject to load or strain which exceeds its regulation capacity.

This is a deceptively simple definition which can explain a large number of physical symptoms of sickness. When the regulation capacity is over-extended the body gets sick. The symptoms are an appropriate reaction to the strain. The symptoms are a survival mechanism which gives the body a chance to outlive the strain, which otherwise could be fatal.

The main forms of stress come in the form of toxins (environmental, stimulants, medicines), deficiencies and mental stress. Toxins put a load on the system, while vitamin and mineral deficiencies reduce the regulation capacity. Mental stress strains the body and at the same time reduces the regulation capacity. Lessening these forms of stress can help to restore your health.

Within a month I recovered to a more normal life. I felt much better and more balanced.

The experience changed my view on health. It made me realize how important it is to reduce the toxic loads on the body. That when the input stress is not managed the body eventually (sometimes sooner than one would like) needs to adjust to the situation by forcing one to slow down, i.e. getting sick or diseased.

This is one reason that I take Kombucha now. I feel like it is helping me lift that toxic load. Besides, after only three months I am surprised to see that my hair is slightly less gray and my skin tone is much better. Since I have changed my view of myself to mind and body I am happy with this development!

THEORIES

What happens when people drink Kombucha tea is described in greater detail in the "What Kombucha Can and Cannot Do" chapter. It is summarized here.

The whole-body approach to health best describes what happens: The tea does not cure anything—the body cures itself. Kombucha seems to help your body do this. There are a number of contributing factors.

DIGESTION involves stomach acid dissolving food and making it ready to be absorbed into the body. Kombucha is somewhat acidic and may help this process, without being so strong as to cause an upset stomach. The tea also contains "people friendly" bacteria which may work with the body's natural bacteria to help finish the digestion process. **Dr. Jim Blechman** in Southern California suggests better digestion could explain people's claims of increased energy, regularity, and improved skin with fewer wrinkles.

But he is far from the first to point out improvement of digestion. In 1928 **Dr. Mollenda** in Germany reported, "In the case of angina, especially when there is a coating of the tonsils, the drink should not merely be used for gargling but for drinking, and that for the destruction of bacteria which reach the stomach through food and drink.... Even though the beverage is acidic, it does not cause any acidic condition in the stomach; it facilitates and noticeably promotes the digestion even of difficult to digest foods. Equally favorable successes after taking Kombucha beverage have also been reached for gouty eczema and for stones in kidneys, urine and gall."

TOXINS are normally removed from the body by the liver and kidneys using glucuronic acid. As we mentioned, this acid binds itself to toxins and allows them to be removed from the body as waste. Since glucuronic acid has been identified in Kombucha tea, the additional supply may allow the body to remove more toxins, which in turn allows the body to function in the normal, natural way it did before toxins built up.

If this is of interest to you, check the books in our reference section by **Artz** and **Osman** (1950) and **Dutton** (1966 and 1980). They follow glucuronic acid from its discovery in 1879 through all the steps of analysis on how detoxification works in the body, drawing on research by experts from many countries.

ANTIBACTERIAL properties of the Kombucha tea have been well documented in studies in the United States (see Hesseltine), Germany and Russia. This might explain the generations-old tradition of grandmothers giving it to family members who suffer from a variety of illnesses.

VITAMINS present in the tea may also contribute to the feeling of general well-being identified by people who use Kombucha.

Millions of people are currently using Kombucha. We hope additional controlled, scientific tests will enable the medical community to fully join the discussion of how to use Kombucha to improve their patients' health. We believe the combination of traditional medicine and Kombucha can produce better results and better overall health. We hope American universities will take on this challenge. It would be good to know the answer.

WHAT IS KOMBUCHA?

Almost everyone seems to know the simple answer to that question. "It's a healthy combination of bacteria and yeast."

But unless people know more than that, rumors will continue to circulate. And some people in the medical community will continue to arch an eyebrow and say, "There isn't anything *known* about it. Just something whipped up in the sink."

So. Take a deep breath. Here we go.

TECHNICAL STUFF

Technically speaking, Kombucha is not a mushroom or fungus. It's a symbiosis (beneficial combination) of healthful bacteria and yeast. The Moscow Central Bacteriological Institute states that it's formed from Bacterium xylinum and nest-like deposits of yeast cells of the genus Saccharomyces. This mixture includes: Saccharomyces ludwigii, Saccharomyces of the apiculatus types, Bacterium xylinoides, Bacterium gluconicum, Schizosaccharomyces pombe, Acetobacter ketogenum, Torula types, Pichia fermentans and other yeasts

They also say that a key ingredient of Kombucha tea is glucuronic acid, which binds up poisons and toxins, both the environmental and metabolic kind, and flushes them out of the body via the kidneys. This is a natural body function which your liver and kidneys do every day, by producing their own glucuronic acid. The tea simply boosts this normal process.

Glucuronic acid is also a building block of a group of important polysaccharides in the body, including hyaluronic acid (a basic component of connective tissue), chondroitin sulfate (a basic component of cartilage), mucoitinsulfuric acid (a building block of the stomach lining and the vitreous humor of the eye), and heparin.

A very small amount of alcohol is produced (about .5%) and the Kombucha tea is lightly carbonated.

The beverage also contains Vitamins B_1, B_2, B_3, B_6, B_{12}, as well as folic acid and L-lactic acid, a substance rarely present in the connective tissue of cancer patients, the lack of which is believed to result in failure of cell respiration and the build-up of undesirable DL-lactic acid in the tissues. Kombucha tea also contains usnic acid which has an antibacterial effect.

That's fairly complex. And it's more of a menu than an understanding of what Kombucha really is. Let's look at it in a more reasonable way.

COMBINATION

Actually, Kombucha is not just a simple combination, in the sense of two things being in the same bowl. It's a symbiotic combination.

A symbiotic combination means the two things depend on each other and help each other survive. To call Kombucha just bacteria or "vinegar plant" would not give the whole picture. To call it just yeast or "fungus" also wouldn't give the full picture.

Yet almost all the articles and news reports about Kombucha fall into that mistake.

The human body is mostly water. Sounds odd, but scientists tell us that's how it is. If a TV station or magazine always referred to people as water (carbonated, distilled, human...?) we'd all enjoy a good laugh.

The same is true of Kombucha. It's not just bacteria, vinegar, yeast or fungus. It is its own living, recognizable thing.

MUSHROOM?

No, it's not a mushroom. People call it that because it looks like one...sort of. The "body" of a Kombucha is a flexible, tough material originally known as Bacterium xylinum. Scientists, as prone to fads as anyone, now call it Acetobacter xylinum.

This "body" was first studied and named by A. J. Brown in England in 1886. He was following up on work done by Louis Pasteur in France a few years earlier. Without the yeasts and bacteria that make this a Kombucha, the "body" is just a vinegar plant. So vinegar is a distant cousin of Kombucha. But the other ingredients in Kombucha give healthy properties to the tea, and a much better taste. Who would want to drink vinegar anyway? Yeech.

FERMENTATION

The basic process that the Kombucha "mushroom" uses to turn sugar, tea and water into Kombucha tea has several steps. The refined white sugar is broken down into simple sugar (i.e. glucose), which is then fermented into alcohol and carbon dioxide. The alcohol is converted into organic acids (acetic, glucuronic, lactic, etc.) and the carbon dioxide becomes carbonation, like you find in a soda drink. Meanwhile the Kombucha mushroom uses the original tea and these organic acids to make a new mushroom. All of this is well documented by other sources such as Günther Frank so we won't repeat it here.

Much of what we just described is the familiar fermentation process. It has been in widespread use ever since cavemen discovered that grain and water sitting in the corner for a couple of weeks could make a nice brew that would blow the pelt off your back.

Making drinks like wine and beer is one use of fermentation—but Kombucha is not very good for that. It uses up the alcohol to make the organic acids and vitamins we described, leaving only .5% in the tea—about the same as non-alcoholic beer.

The other use of fermentation is for preservation of food, and Kombucha is excellent at this—in terms of preserving itself and the tea it makes.

For thousands of years people didn't have the advantages of re-frigeration, freezing, canning bottling or pasteurization. Instead they relied on processes such as drying the food, salting or fermenting it to protect their food from developing dangerous toxins or unhealthy bacteria.

Fermented foods, including cheese, yogurt, kefir, sauerkraut, pickles, certain milks and sourdough types of bread are among many of the foodstuffs protected by this ancient process. This partially explains why naturally fermented Kombucha tea has enjoyed such a long history of safe use.

CLASSIFICATION

We've described a number of things that are distantly related to Kombucha tea, including vinegar, yogurt and kefir. But what is Kombucha? If it's not a bacteria, not a fungus, not a plant—what is it?

Every living thing is identified in a classification system that is used as a common reference in biology and medical studies. It's officially called the taxonomic system, but you can think of it as just the standard classification system.

This system not only defines what each thing is, but what group it is in and how that group is related to all other living things.

In these classifications, virtually everything is divided into one of five groups. Those groups have Latin names, but in plain English they are:

ANIMALS   BACTERIA   FUNGUS   ALGAE   PLANTS

These groups are called kingdoms. You've probably heard people refer to the animal kingdom. This is where the expression comes from.

These kingdoms are then divided into several levels of smaller groups. This is similar to countries being divided into states, then states divided into counties.

Each kingdom is divided into groups called a "phylum." Each phylum is divided into several "class" groups, and so on. The different levels of classification for living things are shown here:

		Examples	
		Human Being	White Oak
Kingdom	General	Animalia	Plantae
Phylum		Chordata	Magnoliophyta
Class		Mamalia	Magnoliopsida
Order		Primates	Fagales
Family		Hominidae	Fagaceae
Genus		*Homo*	*Quercus*
Species	Specific	*Homo sapiens*	*Quercus alba*

With that general picture, we need to get into some details to show exactly what Kombucha is. It will be important that we're able to distinguish between the five kingdoms, so let's look at them in a little more detail.

Animalia—All animals. Multi-cell organisms that have well-defined shape, can move voluntarily, actively acquire food, and have sensory nerve systems.

Monera—All bacteria. Single cell organisms that have no nucleus, typically reproduce by budding or fission, and have a nutritional mode of absorption, photosynthesis or chemosynthesis, including bacteria and blue-green algae.

Fungi—All fungus. Single or multi-cell organisms that have a nucleus, which live by decomposing and absorbing the organic material in which they grow, including mushrooms, molds, and yeasts.

Protista—All algae except blue-green. Single cell organisms that have a nucleus and are free-living or aggregated into colonies, including protozoa and all algae except blue-green.

Plantae—All plants. Multi-cell organisms that typically produce their own food from inorganic matter by photosynthesis and have cell walls containing cellulose.

By these definitions, we see that symbiotic combinations of living things from two different kingdoms require a specific classification, since they don't fall into one kingdom or the other.

LICHEN

A familiar example of this is lichen. Lichen is a symbiotic combination of fungus and algae having a green, gray, yellow, brown or black "body" that grows in leaf-like, crust-like or branching form on rocks, trees, etc. It is classified in its own family group between the "Fungi" and "Protista" kingdoms.

KOMBUCHA

Following that precedent, the same should apply to Kombucha. It should be classified into its own family group between the "Fungi" and "Monera" kingdoms.

The larger family to which Kombucha belongs would be defined as follows. "A complex organism composed of bacteria in symbiotic union with yeast, existing in a liquid or solid medium, and usually growing in the presence of a sugar dissolved in water."

It is proposed that the scientific term for this family be "stadelen," in honor of Dr. Eduard Stadelmann who has been instrumental in advancing Kombucha research in Europe and the United States for over 35 years.

Clearly, Kombucha is in this family. But other things may be found to exist in this category besides Kombucha—other combinations of bacteria and yeast which have other properties and characteristics.

So we should define a specific genus called "Kombucha," as follows. "A complex organism composed of Acetobacter xylinum in symbiotic union with yeast of the genus Saccharomyces, and possibly other bacteria or yeasts, usually growing in layers of cellulose formed by the bacteria with nest-like deposits of yeast, in the presence of a sugar dissolved in a tea."

Good. We're almost done. The last step is to recognize that within the group called Kombucha there are likely to be several different varieties. Something which has traveled all over the world and been passed down from generation to generation is very likely to have adapted into several different types (species).

Most of the Kombuchas in the United States are descendants of the excellent species cultivated by Betsy Pryor. For this reason, Sandy Holst suggests that when sufficient laboratory analysis has been done on this particular species to identify how it might differ from others (in Italy, for example), that **this predominant U.S. species be named Kombucha pryor.**

REFERENCES

WHERE TO FIND A KOMBUCHA

There are many places you can get Kombucha mushrooms across the United States. If you ask people where you work or put a message on the local market bulletin board, you're likely to find someone who can give you one. Anybody with a Kombucha gets a baby mushroom every week or ten days and is usually happy to share with someone who's interested.

Normally they'll insist you have it free. You often find that people who use Kombucha feel a small miracle fell into their life, and are happy to share their experience.

If for some reason that route doesn't get you a mushroom, you can contact one of the commercial growers across the country.

Betsy Pryor, in addition to appearing on television and radio, and speaking to live groups about Kombucha, is the founder of Laurel Farms, widely recognized as the leader among American growers. They charge a fee for their mushrooms, but make special arrangements for people suffering from serious illnesses who are in financial need.

Whether your mushroom comes from a friend or a grower, try to learn if they follow the clean "growing" method described in this book. You need a healthy mushroom to get good results.

INFORMATION

If you have specific questions or want information on obtaining a Kombucha mushroom, send a stamped, self-addressed envelope to:

Ms. Betsy Pryor
Laurel Farms
P.O. Box 7405
Studio City, California 91614

Here are two other reliable sources of information on the Kombucha mushroom. Be sure to enclose a self-addressed envelope and international postage voucher for reply.

Mr. Günther Frank
Genossenschafts Strasse 10
75217 Birkenfeld
Germany

Ms. Rosina Fasching
Post Box 98
A-9021 Klagenfurt
Austria

INTERNET

Another outstanding source is the **Internet**, if you're interested in cyber-talking with people who know about Kombucha. As a good starting place, we recommend the on-line discussion groups in the popular Internet-access services:

On **Prodigy**, access the Health Bulletin Board. We saw a lively discussion there in the topic area of Holistic Medicine and the specific subject of Kombucha.

America-On-Line has a bulletin board (or "forum") called Longevity which had a good discussion on Kombucha. Some of the individuals kept in touch afterward and exchanged personal e-mail and experiences with Kombucha.

WORLD WIDE WEB

This is the fastest growing part of the Net, and Kombucha pages seem to be growing faster than almost any other subject. If you log on, plan to stay a while to see them all. We recommend that you start with the Kombucha Home Page maintained by Jim Sease, one of the pioneers in bringing Kombucha on-line. You can find it at:

http://www.sease.com/kombucha/index.html

KOMBUCHA MAILING LIST

If you're really into Kombucha and would like to be involved in one of the most stimulating and challenging mailing lists on the Net, have we got the one for you! Once you subscribe to the list (it's free—just submit your e-mail name and you're on.) expect to get ten or twenty messages every day. All on Kombucha. You can respond to any of them or just "lurk" and read what's going on.

It works like this. When you "post" a message (by sending an e-mail to the list address) it automatically goes to everyone on the list. Any number of people might respond with information, their experiences or more questions—and on it goes.

If the volume of mail overwhelms your mailbox, you can request your mail come in the form of a "digest." It's one e-mail, sent each day, containing all the messages sent to the list that day. This is definitely recommended unless you have a lot of time to keep up with all the mail.

Here's what you need to know to take this wild ride on the waves of Kombucha e-mail.

1. **Subscribe to the list.** Send a message to:

   kombucha-request@shore.net

   In the body of the message type:
   subscribe
   end

2. **Or subscribe to the digest.** Send a message to:

   kombucha-digest-request@shore.net

   In the body of the message type:

   subscribe
   end

3. **Check your e-mail** the next day to see the current river of Kombucha info that's flowing past.

4. **Send your first e-mail**, jump in and swim. The water's fine!

   To: kombucha@shore.net

5. For future use, **get the list of commands** you can use with this list. Send a message to:

   kombucha-request@shore.net

   In the body of the message type:
   help
   end

6. A very important command: If you get exhausted from the volume of Kombucha info, and many people do, here's how you **get off the list.** If you're on the basic list, send a message to:

kombucha-request@shore.net

In the body of the message type:

unsubscribe
end

If you're on the digest list, send a message to:

kombucha-digest-request@shore.net

In the body of the message type:

unsubscribe
end

MORE INTERNET

For a source of files and info on Kombucha other than the World Wide Web, we recommend you start with the Kombucha Tea Cider Gopher sponsored by Arizona State University at:

enuxsa.eas.asu.edu 6600

Cyber-surf's up. Catch a wave!

BOOKS AND ARTICLES

Abele, Johann (In German): Teepilz Kombucha bei Diabetes? Der Naturarzt. vol. 110, no.12:31. (Kombucha Tea Mushroom for Diabetes?) 1988

Arauner, E. (In German): Der japanische Teepilz. Dtsch. Essigindustrie. vol. 33, no.2:11-12. (The Japanese Tea Mushroom) 1929

Artz, Neal E., Osman, Elizabeth M. (In English): Biochemistry of Glucuronic Acid. New York Academic Press. New York. 1950

Bacinskaya, A.A. (In Russian): O rasprostranenii "cainogo kvassa" i Bacterium xylinum Brown. Zurnal Microbiologii. I:73-85. Petrograd. (On the distribution of "tea kvass" and Bacterium xylinum Brown.) 1914

Barbancik, G.F. (In Russian): Cainii grib i ego lecebnye svoistva. Izdame Tretye. Omsk: Omskoe oblastnoe kniznoe izdatelstvo. (The tea fungus and its therapeutic properties.) 1954

Bazarewski, S. (In German): Über den sogenannten "Wunderpilz" in den baltischen Provinzen. Correspondenzblatt Naturforscher-Verein. 57:61-69. Riga. (Concerning the "Miracle Mushroom" in the Baltic Provinces.) 1915

Bing, M. (In German): Heilwirkung des "Kombuchaschwammes". Umschau. 32:913-914. (Healing properties of the "Kombucha sponge.") 1928

Bing, M. (In German): Der Symbiont Bacterium xylinum— Schizosaccharomyces Pombe als Therapeutikum. Die medizinische Welt. 2(42):1576-1577. (The Therapeutic Symbiosis of Bacterium Xylinum—Schizosaccharomyces Pombe.) 1928

Bing, M. (In German): Zur Kombucha-frage. Die Umschau. 33(6):118-119. (On the Kombucha Question.) 1929

Brown, A.J. (In English): On an acetic Ferment which forms Cellulose. Journal of the Chemical Society. 49:432-439. London. 1886

Bruker, M.O. (In German): Antwort auf Leseranfrage zu Kombucha. Der Naturarzt Vol. 108 11:14. (Answer to reader's question about Kombucha). 1986.

Chopra, Deepak (In English): Ageless Body, Timeless Mind. Harmony Books. New York. 1993.

Danielova, L.T. (In Russian): Bakteriostaticeskoe i baktericidnoe svoistvo nastoia "cainogo griba". Trudy Yerevanskogo zooverterinarnogo Instituta. 11:31-41. (The bacteriostatic and bactericidal properties of the "tea fungus" infusion.) 1949

Danielova, L.T. (In Russian): K morfologii "cainogo griba". Trudy Yerevanskogo zooverterinarnogo Instituta. 17:201-216. (Morphology of the "tea fungus.") 1954

Danielova, L.T. (In Russian): Biologiceskie osobennosti cainogo griba. Trudy Yerevanskogo zooverterinarnogo Instituta. 23:159-164. (The special biological characteristics of the tea fungus.) 1959

Dinslage, E., Ludorff, W. (In German): Der "indische Teepilz". Zeitschrift für Untersuchung der Lebensmittel. 53:458-467. (The "Indian Tea Mushroom.") 1927

Dutton, G.J. (In English): Glucuronic Acid. (GJD ed.) Academic Press. New York. 1966

Dutton, G.J. (In English): Glucuronidation of Drugs and Other Compounds. CRC Press, Boca Raton. 1980

Fasching, Rosina (Translated from German): Tea Fungus Kombucha, the Natural Remedy and its Significance in Cases of Cancer and other Metabolic Diseases. Publisher: Wilhelm Ennsthaler, A-4402, Steyr, Austria. 1985

Filho, L.X., Paulo, M.Q., Pareira, E.C., Vicente, C. Phenolics from tea fungus analyzed by high performance liquid chromatography. Phyton (Buenos Aires). vol. 45, no.2:187-191. 1985

Flexner, Stuart B. (In English): The Random House Dictionary of the English Language, Second Edition, Unabridged. (SBF ed.) Random House. New York. 1987

Flück, V., Steinegger, E. (In German): Eine neue Hefekomponente des Teepilzes. Scientia pharmaceutica (Vienna). 25:43-44. (A New Yeast Component of Tea Mushrooms.) 1957

Fontana, J.D., Franco, V.C., DeSouza, S.J., Lyra, I.N., DeSouza, A.M. (In English): Nature of Plant Stimulators in the Production of Acetobacter xylinum ("Tea Fungus") Biofilm Used in Skin Therapy. Applied Biochemistry and Biotechnology (Curitiba, PR, Brazil). Vol. 28/29:341-351. 1991

Foster, Daniel (In English): The Mushroom That Ate LA. Los Angeles Magazine. vol. 39, no.11:118-124. Los Angeles. 1994

Frank, Günther (Translated from German): Kombucha, healthy beverage and natural remedy from the Far East, its correct preparation and use. Publisher: Wilhelm Ennsthaler, A-4402 Steyr, Austria. 1991

Funke, Hans (In German): Der Teepilz Kombucha. Natur & Heilen. 64:509–513. (The Tea Mushroom Kombucha.) 1987

Gadd, C.H. (In English): Tea Cider. Tea Quarterly (Talawakelle, Sri Lanka). 6:48–53. 1933

Gordienko, M. (In German): Review of a report (in Russian) by **Utkin, L.** Zbl. Bakt. 98,II:359. 1937

Haehn, H., Engel, M. (In German): Über die Bildung von Milchsäure durch Bacterium xylinum. Milchsäuregärung durch Kombucha. Zentralblatt für Bakteriologie, Mikrobiologie und Hygiene. II:182-185. (Concerning the formation of lactic acid through Bacterium xylinum. Latic acid formation through Kombucha.) 1929

Hahmann, C. (In German): Über Drogen und Drogenverfäl–schungen. Apotheker-Zeitung. vol. 44, no. 37:561-563. 1929

Harms, H. (In German): Der japanische Teepilz. Therapeutische Berichte, Leverkusen. p. 498–500. 1927

Henneberg, W. (In German): Zur Kenntnis der Schnellessig-und Weinessigbakterien. Zentralblatt für Bakteriologie. vol. 17, no. 25:789-804. 1907

Henneberg, W. (In German): Handbuch der Gärungsbakteriologie, Vol. 2 (Spezielle Pilzkunde, unter besonderer Berücksichtigung der Hefe-, Essigund Milchsäurebakterien), 2nd edition. Verlag Paul Parey. Berlin 1926.

Hensler, P.O. (In German): Alles über Kombucha. Stutensee. (All About Kombucha.) 1989

Hermann, S. (In German): Über die sogenannte Kombucha. Biochemische Zeitschrift. 192:176-199. (About that which is called Kombucha.) 1928

Hermann, S. (In German): Die sogenannte "Kombucha." Umschau. 33:841-844. (That which is called Kombucha.) 1929

Hermann, S., Fodor, N. (In German): C-Vitamin-(l-Ascorbinsäure)-Bildung durch eine Symbiose von Essigbakterien und Hefen. Biochemische Z. vol.276, nos.5-6:323-325. (C-Vitamin {Ascorbic Acid} Formation through a Symbiosis of Vinegar Bacteria and Yeasts.) 1935

Hesseltine, Clifford W. (In English): A Millenium of Fungi, Food and Fermentation. Mycologia. 57:149-197. 1965

Irion, H. (In German): Fungus japonicus, Fungojapon Kombucha—Indisch-japanischer Teepilz. (IH ed.) Lehrgang für Drogistenfachschulen, Vol. 2 (Botanik/Drogenkunde), 4th edition. Verlagsgesellschaft Rudolf Müller. Eberswalde-Berlin-Leipsig. (Training Course for Pharmaceutical Technical Colleges.) 1944

Kaminski, Anette (In German): Ärzte: Pilz heilt Frauenleiden. Bild der Frau No. 2. Axel Springer Verlag. Hamburg. 1988

Kasevnik, L.L. (In Russian): Biohimia Vitamina C. Soobscenie III. O sposobnosti japonskogo cainogo griba sintezirovat' Vitamin C.—Bull. exp. Biol. i Med (Moscow) vol.3, no.1:87-88. [See Schwaibold, N., for a review of this report.] (The biochemistry of vitamin C. 3rd report: The ability of the Japanese tea fungus to produce vitamin C.) 1937

Kobert, R. (In German): Der Kwass—ein unschädliches billiges Volkgetränk. 2nd edition. Haale a. d. Saale. 1913

Köhler, Valentin (In German): Glukuronsäure macht Krebspatienten Mut. Ärztliche Praxis. 33:887. (Glucuronic Acid Gives Cancer Patients Hope.) 1981

Köhler, Valentin, Köhler, J. (In German): Glukuronsäure als ökologische Hilfe. In the book: Sofortheilung des Waldes, Vol. 1, 2nd edition. (H. Kaegelmann ed.) Verlag zur heilen Welt. Windecke-Rosbach. (Glucuronic acid as an ecological aid.) 1985

Konovalov, I.N., Litvinov, M.A., Zakman, L.M. (In Russian): Izmenenie prirody i fiziologiceskii osobennostei cainogo griba (Medusomyces gisevii Lindau) v zavisimosti ot uslovii kultivirovania. Bit Zurnal (Moscow). vol. 44, no. 3:346-349. (Changes in the nature and physiological properties of the tea fungus (Medusomyces gisevii Lindau) regarding the requirements of the culture medium.) 1959

Körner, Helmut (In German): Der Teepilz Kombucha. Der Naturarzt. vol. 108,no. 5:14-16. (The Tea Mushroom Kombucha.) 1987

Körner, Helmut (In German): Kombucha-Zubereitung wurde von Sportmedizinern getestet. Natura-med (Neckarsulm). vol.4, no.10:592. (Kombucha preparation tested by sports physicians.) 1989

Kozaki, M., Koizumi, A., Kitagara, K. Microorganism of Zoogleal Mats Formed on Tea Decoction. J. Food Hyg. Soc. Japan. 13:89-96. 1972

Kraft, M.M. (In French): Le Champignon de Thé. Nova Hedwigia. vol. 1, nos. 3-4:297-304. (The Tea Mushroom.) 1959

Kreger-van Rij, N.J.W. (In English): The Yeasts: A Taxonomic Study. Elsevier. Amsterdam. 1984

Lakowitz, N. (In German): Teepilz und Teekwass. Apotheker-Zeitung. 43:298-300. 1928

Leskov, A.I. (In Russian): Novye svedenya o cainom gribe. Feldser i Akuerka (Moscow) vol. 23, no. 10:47-48. (New information about the tea fungus.) 1958

Lindau, G. (In German): Über Medusomyceš Gisevii, eine neue Gattung und Art der Hefepilze. Ber. dt. bot. Ges. 31:243-248. (Concerning Medusomyces Gisevii, a New Genus and Spieces of Yeast Mushroom.) 1913

Lindner, P. (In German): Die vermeintliche neue Hefe Medusomyces Gisevii. Ber. dt. bot. Ges. 31:364-368. 1913

Lindner, P. (In German): Über Teekwass und Teekwasspilze. Mikrokosmos. 11:93-98. 1917

List, P.H., Hufschmidt, W. (In German): Basische Pilzinhaltsstoffe. 5. Mitteilung über biogene Amine und Aminosäuren des Teepilzes. Pharm. Zentralhalle. 98:593-598. 1959

Löwenheim, H. (In German): Über den indischen Teepilz. Apotheker-Zeitung. 42:148-149. (Concerning the Indian Tea Mushroom.) 1927

Mann, Ulrike (In German): Verblüffend—ein Pilz kuriert den Darm. Bild und Funk No. 35. Burda GmbH, Offenburg. (Amazing—a mushroom heals the intestines.) 1988

Marshak, Alfred (In English): A Crystalline Antibacterial Substance From the Lichen *Ramalina Reticulata*. Public Health Reports. Vol. 62, no. 1:3-19. 1947

Matern, S., Bock, K.W., Gerok, W. (In English): Advances in Glucuronide Conjugation. (SM, KWB, WG ed.) MTP Press, Lancaster, United Kingdom. 1985

Meixner, A. (In German): Pilze selber züchten. Aarau (Switzerland). (Cultivating mushrooms yourself.) 1989

Merck Index (In English): Glucuronic Acid, p. 701. Usnic Acid, p. 1557. Eleventh Edition. 1989

Mollenda, L. (In German): Kombucha, ihre Heilbedeutung und Züchtung. Deutsche Essigindustrie. vol. 32, no. 27:243-244. (Kombucha, its healing properties and cultivation.) 1928

Mulder, D. (In English): A revival of tea cider. Tea Quarterly (Talawakelle, Sri Lanka). 32:48-53. 1961

Naumova, E.K. (In Russian): Meduzin—Novoe antibioticeskoe vescestvo, obrazumoe Medusomyces Gisevii. In: Vtoraya naucnaya Konferencia sanitarnogigieniceskogo fakulteta. 28-29 Aprelia 1949. Avtoreferati. p. 20-23. Kazan: Kazanskii gosudarstvenni medicinskii Institut. (Meduzin—a new antibiotic substance formed by Medusomyces Gisevii. In: second Scientific Conference of the Faculty of Health and Hygiene, April 28-29, 1949. Report p. 20-23. The Kazan State Medical Institute.) 1949

Parker, S.B. (In English): Synopsis and Classification of Living Organisms. McGraw Hill. New York. 1982

Paula Gomes, A. de (In Portuguese): Observações sobre a utilização de Zymomonas mobilis (Lindner) Kluyver et van Niel, 1936. (Thermobacterium mobile, Lindner 1928; Pseudomonas linderi Kluyver et Hoppenbrouwers, 1931), na Térapeutica Humana. Revista Instituto de Antibióticos (Pernambuco, Brazil). 2:77-81. 1959

People Magazine Staff (In English): Yeast Meets West. People Magazine. vol. 43, no. 6:192. 1995

Popiel, L.v. (In German): Zur Selbstherstellung von Essig. Pharmaz. Post (Vienna). vol.50, no.80:757-758. (On making vinegar oneself.) 1917

Reiss, Jürgen (In German): Der Teepilz und seine Stoffwechselprodukte. Deutsche Lebenmittel-Rundschau. vol.83, no.9:286-290. (The tea mushroom and its metabolic components.) 1987

Roots, H. (In Estonian): Teeseeneleotise Ravitoimest. Noukogude eesti tervishoid (Tallin, Estonia). 2:55-57. (The curative powers of the tea fungus.) 1959

Sakaryan, G.A., Danielova, L.T. (In Russian): Antibioticeskie svoistva nastoia griba Medusomyces gisevii (cainogo griba). Soobscenie 1. Trudy Yerevanskogo zooveterinarnogo Insttuta. 10:33-45. (The antibiotic capacities of the infusion of Medusomyces gisevii (tea fungus). 1st Report.) 1948

Schröder, H. (In German): Teepilz und japanische Kristalle. Deine Gesundheit (Berlin). 7:29-30. 1989

Schwaibold, N. (In German): Review of a report (in Russian) by **Kasevkik, L.D.** Chem. Zbl. II:2860. 1937

Silva, R.L. de, Saravanapavan, T.V. (In English): Tea cider—a potential winner. Tea Quarterly (Talawakelle, Sri Lanka). 39:37-40. 1969

Sklenar, Rudolf (In German): Ein in der Iris sichtbarer Test für eine Stoffwechselstörung, kontrolliert an Hand von Dunkelfelduntersuchungen des Blutes nach Scheller. Erfahrungsheilkunde. vol.13, no. 3. 1964

Sklenar, Rudolf (In German): Krebsdiagnose aus dem Blut und die Behandlung von Krebs, Präkanzerosen und sonstigen Stoffwechselkrankheiten mit der Kombucha und Colipräparaten. Published by Fasching. Klagenfurt. (Cancer Diagnosis From Blood and the Treatment of Cancer and Pre-Cancerous Ailments by Means of Kombucha and Colicines.) 1983

Smuts, J.C. (In English): Holism and Evolution. MacMillan. New York. 1926

Stadelmann, Eduard (In German): Der Teepilz—Eine Literaturzusammenstellung. Sydowia, Ann. mycolog. Ser. II. II:380-388. (The Tea Mushroom—A Compilation of Literature.) 1957

Stadelmann, Eduard (In German): Der Teepilz un seine antibiotische Wirkung. Zentralblatt Bakt. I. Abt. Ref. 180:401-435. (The Tea Mushroom and its Antibacterial Action.) 1961

Stark, J.B., Walter, E.D., Owens, H.S. (In English): Method of Isolation of Usnic Acid from *Ramalina reticulata*. Journal of the American Chemical Society. 72:1819-1820. 1950

Steiger, K.E., Steinegger, E. (In German): Über den Teepilz. Pharmaceutica Acta Helvetiae. 32:133-154. (Concerning the Tea Mushroom.) 1957

Sukiasyan, A.O. (In Russian): Vliyanie faktorov vnesnei sredy i istocnikov pitanya na nakoplenie antibioticeskii vescestv v kulture "cainogo griba". Soobscenie 1. Izucenie razlicnii fiziko-mehaniceskii vozodeistvii. Trudy Yerevanskogo zooveterinarnogo Instituta. 17:229-235. (The influence of culture milieu factors and nutrient sources on the accumulation of antibacterial substances in "tea fungus" cultures. 1st Report. The investigation of various physico-mechanical influences.) 1954

Tea Export Bureau, Batavia (In English): Tea cider—a new drink in Java. Tea Quarterly (Talawakelle, Sri Lanka). 5:126-127. 1932

Utkin, L. (In Russian): O novom mikroorganizme iz gruppy uksusnyi bakterii. Mikrobiologia (Moscow). vol.6, no.4:421-434. [See **Gordienko, M.** for a review of this report.] (On a new micro-organism of the acetic acid group.) 1937

Valentin, H. (In German): Über die Verwendung des indischen Teepilzes und seine Gewinnung in trockener Form. Apotheker-Zeitung 43:1533-1536. 1928

Valentin, H. (In German): Wesentliche Bestandteile der Gärungsprodukte in den durch Pilztätigkeit gewonnenen Hausgetränken sowie die Verbreitung der letzteren. Apotheker-Zeitung. 45:1464-1465 and 1477-1478. (Essential components of fermentation products in the beverage gained by mushroom activity as well as its distribution.) 1930

Waldeck, H. (In German): Der Teepilz. Pharmazeutische Zentralhalle. 68:789-790. (The Tea Mushroom.) 1927

Wiechowski, W. (In German): Welche Stellung soll der Arzt zur Kombuchafrage einnehmen? Beiträge zur ärztlichen Fortbildung. 6:2-10. Prague. (What Position Should a Doctor Take on the Kombucha Question?) 1928

Winberg-Nielsen, K. (In Danish): Biopati—en vej til sundhed. Narayana Press. Gylling, Denmark. (Biopathy—a way to health.) 1982

Yermolayeva, Z.V., Vaisberg, G.E., Afanaseyeva, T.I., Givenstal, N.I. (In Russian): O stimulyacii nekotorii antibakterialnii faktorov v organizme zitvotnii. Antibiotiki (Moscow). 3(6):46-50. (The stimulation of specific antibacterial factors in the animal organism.) 1958

Special thanks to Professor Stadelmann for many references, and to Lisa Hornung for helping to translate them.

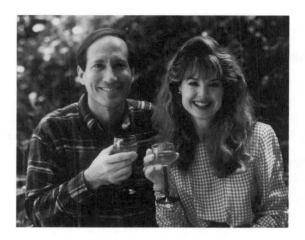

Sanford (Sandy) Holst & Betsy Pryor

THE LAST WORD

This book was carefully prepared using all the facts and information available to us about this remarkable health trend in the United States. We drew upon many previous studies and publications from other countries, which are gratefully acknowledged.

Since water, climate, cleanliness and other things affect the "growing" process, we can't guarantee the quality of the tea you make. But it's been grown for hundreds of years under a wide range of conditions, so you'll probably do fine.

Everyone's interested in their health and making the right decisions. We've tried to give the best possible information to help you, but obviously we can't make recommendations about anyone's particular medical case. Check with your health care provider.

Enjoy. Be happy. And healthy.

Betsy Pryor
Sanford Holst

INDEX

A

Acidity, 20, 48, 66, 127
Acne, 23, 39
AIDS/HIV, 14, 40–42, 71
Allergy, 53
America On Line, 139
Animals, 109
Antibacterial, 68, 73
Applying to skin, 108
Arizona, 40, 42, 48
Arkansas, 27, 102
Arthritis, 50, 59
Asia, 115–117
Asthma, 53

B

Baby mushrooms, 15, 78,
    82–86, 91–96, 137
Bacteria, 20, 67–68, 129–135
Betsy Pryor Method, 77, 97–
    99
Bladder, 57
Blechman, Jim, 127
Bottled, 105
Bowl, 65, 78
Bruker, M., 20, 142
Bubbles, 89

C

California, 19, 25, 35, 39,
    41, 45, 47, 53, 56–58, 108
Cancer, 17, 27, 42–45
Candida, 38–40
Celebrities, 11, 24, 55
Centers for Disease Control,
    69–70
Ceramic, 63, 78
Cheesecloth, 79
Chemotherapy, 43–45
China, 115
Chopra, Deepak, 26, 142
Chronic fatigue, 45–48
Claims, 11, 17
Classification, 132–135
Clean, 64, 83
Cloth, 79, 84
Complexion, 23
Contaminant, 61–68, 92
Coolidge, Rita, 11, 55
Cornell University, 121
Crystal, 63, 78

D

DeHaan, Roger, 110–113
Derry, Joan, 14, 120

Detoxify, 70, 78, 127
Diabetes, 30–34, 59
Diarrhea, 42
Digestion, 48–50, 127
Doctor, 33, 65
Dutton, Geoffrey, 127, 143

E

Eating mushroom, 60, 104
Energy, 15, 19–20
Europe, 117–120
Evans, Linda, 11

F

Fairchild, Morgan, 11
Farrell, Sharon, 11
Fasching, Rosina, 120, 138
Fatigue, 45–48
FDA, 63, 67, 69
Fermentation, 131–132
Fibromyalgia, 46–47
First-time drinkers, 103
Florida, 60, 108
Flu, 53
Frank, Günther, 119, 131, 138
Freezing, 92
Fruit flies, 79, 84, 88
Funnel, 79

G

Gates, Jeffrey, 121
Georgia, 28, 45, 53
Germany, 119, 122–123, 127
Getting mushroom, 82, 95, 137–138

Giving mushroom, 93–94
Glucuronic acid, 70, 127, 130
Growing, 83–88, 98–99
Gulf War Syndrome, 57

H

Hair, 15, 24–26
Hannah, Daryl, 11
Harvest, 86–87, 94
Health food store, 105–106
Heller, Richard, 121
Heller, Rachael, 121
Hemorrhoids, 56
Heparin, 56–57, 130
Herbal tea, 65, 79, 82, 94–95
Hernia, 56
Hesseltine, 73, 121, 145
Holes, 90
Holistic, 19, 110, 123–126
Holst, Sanford, 10, 26, 55, 135, 153
Honey, 82

I

Illinois, 57
Indiana, 50
Indigestion, 48–50, 127
Internet, 138–141
Iowa, 24, 62, 69–70
Italy, 119, 122

J

Japan, 116–117, 122
Jar, 78, 89
Jetlag, 55
Juices, 102

K

Kargasok, 117
Kvass, 71, 122

L

Landau, Martin, 24
Liberia, 13

M

Madonna, 11
Making tea, 77–99
Massachusetts, 22
Medications, 27, 54, 63, 65, 107
Metal, 80–83
Michigan, 50, 56
Microwave, 91
Migraine, 50–53
Minnesota, 121
Mold, 38, 64, 66–67, 73, 84, 90
Mollenda, L., 127, 148
Morocco, 68–69
Mother mushroom, 86–88, 91
Multiple sclerosis, 34–37, 58
Mycological Society of America, 73, 121

N

Names for beverage, 122
Names for mushroom, 122
Nausea, 41, 106
Neighbor, 15, 48, 92, 96
New Mexico, 55

New York, 19, 49, 56
North Carolina, 30

O

Ohio, 26, 34, 48, 109

P

Pain, 50–53, 57
Pan/pot, 81
Plants, 83, 90, 109
Pennsylvannia, 31
Plastic, 63, 78, 82
Povitch, Maury, 29
Prodigy, 138
Protection against contamination, 66–68
Pryor, Betsy, 10, 13, 29, 109, 120, 138, 153

Q

Quantity of tea, 29, 88, 101

R

Reagan, Ronald, 11
Reiss, Jürgen, 20, 148
Rheumatism, 50–53
Rubber band, 80
Rumors, 68–74
Russel, Graham, 11
Russia, 28, 60, 117–119, 122

S

Safety, 9, 61–75
Seniors, 15, 19, 25, 32, 56, 58–60

Separating mushrooms, 86, 103
Sex, 30
Shred, 90
Side effects, 106–107
Skin, 20–24, 26, 42, 58, 108, 127
Sklenar, Rudolf, 119, 149
Smell, 83–85
Smuts, Jan Christian, 123, 149
Sore throat, 53–55
Spoon, 80
Stadelmann, Eduard, 71, 121, 135, 150, 151
Stalin, 119
Steinkraus, Keith, 121
Storing tea, 103–105
Stress, 48–50
Studies, 106, 111, 119–121, 127
Substitutions, 82
Sugar, 19, 30, 80
Sunlight, 85
Switzerland, 119, 121

T

Tape, 84, 99
Taste, 102–105
Tea, Black, 79
 - Green, 79
 - Herbal, 65, 82, 94–95
 - Old, 83, 84
Temperature, 85, 91–92
Texas, 23, 34, 56
Theories, 126–128
Thin, 91

Time, Growing, 86, 102–103
 Storing, 103–105
Tomlin, Lily, 11

U

Ulcers, 48–49
United States, 120–121
Usnic acid, 68, 130

V

Vacation, 92
Valentine, Tom, 120
Vibration, 91
Vinegar, 73, 130
Virginia, 117
Vitamins, 128, 130

W

Washington, 115
Water, 81
Weight, 15, 26–28, 49, 58, 101
Wilen, Joan, 54
Wilen, Lydia, 54
Winberg-Nielsen, Kurt, 125–126
Wisconsin, 58
World Health Organization, 40
World Wide Web, 139
Wydoff, Boris, 28
Wyoming, 41

Y

Yeast, 38–40, 104, 129

Get your own copy of
KOMBUCHA PHENOMENON

⟨ Or send one to a friend ⟩

It's as easy as . . .

1 Tell us where to send it:

Name _____

Address _____

City _____ State ___ Zip _____

If it's a gift, fill in your name:

It's a gift from

_____

2 And send a check or money order for

Book 11.95
Shipping 1.90
$ 13.85

California residents add sales
tax for a total of **$ 14.85**

3 To: Sierra Sunrise Books
14622 Ventura Blvd, Suite 800
Sherman Oaks, CA 91403

(Allow 2–4 weeks for delivery)
(You may copy this order form)   BOOK-2